IN INTIMATE DETAIL

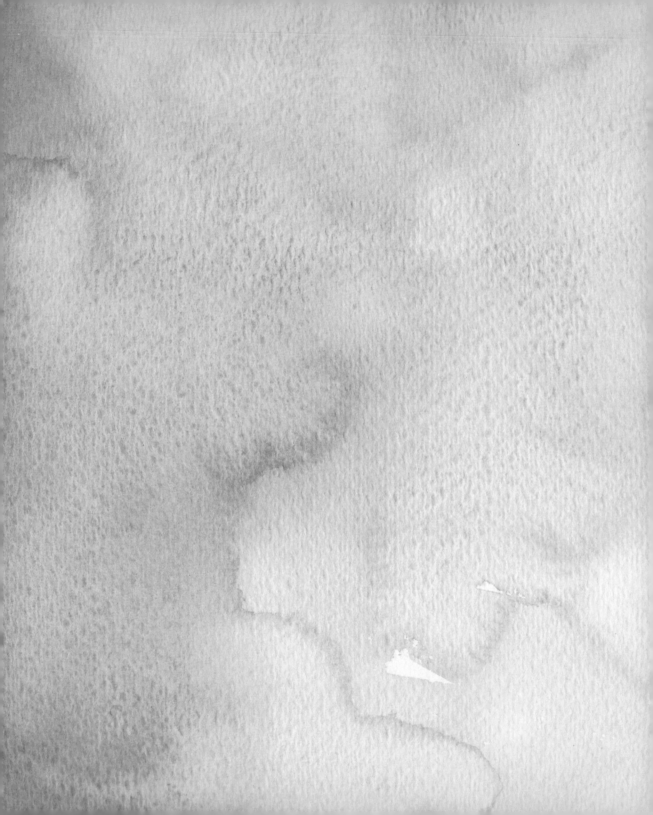

IN INTIMATE DETAIL

How to Choose, Wear, and Love Lingerie

Cora Harrington

**Foreword by
Dita Von Teese**

Illustrations by Sandy Wirt

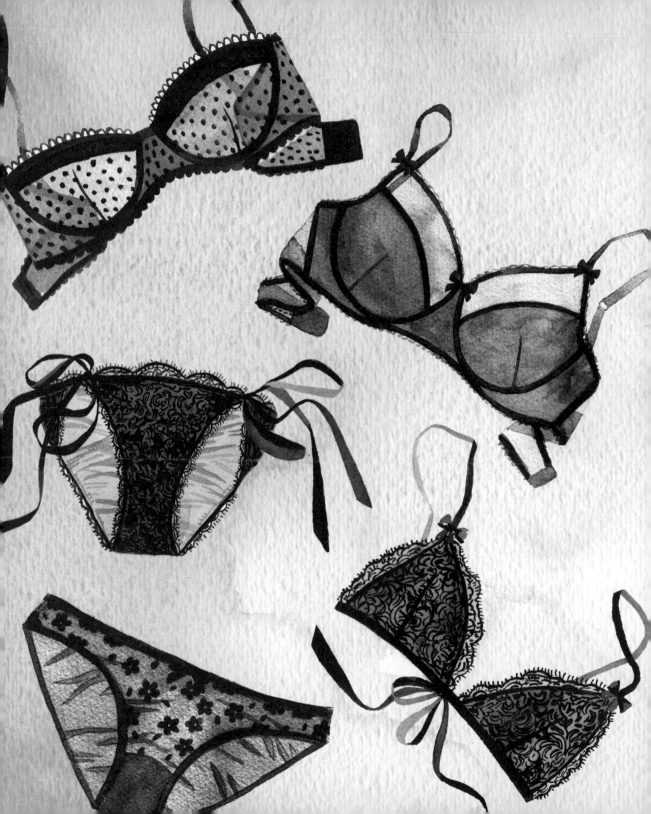

CONTENTS

Foreword

Why wear lingerie? Given my longstanding and intimate relationship with this body of garments—from my first job in a lingerie boutique to a career being tight-laced into corsets only to sling them off, and as designer of my very own signature lines of lingerie and full-fashioned stockings—well, it's a question that comes up more often than not.

Singles will confide in me that they don't bother since they have no one special in their life to impress. Those with a special someone in their lives dismiss any need to bother because they are "past" that stage. Then there are those who believe their figure doesn't deserve pretty lingerie. Seriously? Flying solo or not, zaftig or gamine, you should never stuff your sensuality in a drawer for another lifetime. Lingerie is an opportunity! And not how you might think. Lingerie offers a chance to honor your *self* every day.

I like to say that lingerie allows for the seduction of self. You are the first to experience that pretty lace bra or slip into those silken knickers. You might also be the only one in on the secret under that black dress, concealing a ravishing crimson camisole you selected even if no one would ever be the wiser. Beautiful lingerie should not be limited as an instrument to catch a lover. It is a signal that you love yourself enough to take out the good stuff and feel special even on the most mundane of days. To get to this point takes a bit of practice, of course. It takes patience, at least initially, to slip into seamed stockings and hook them into place. Or to zero in on a cup shape that looks as good as it feels. But soon, these rituals will feel effortless, even fulfilling.

My own love affair with lingerie began when I was a young girl. I was transfixed by the starlets clad in slinky negligees and marabou-trimmed robes appearing in the old movies playing on Saturday afternoon TV. My first job was in a lingerie boutique, where I learned to properly fit a bra. I shopped for vintage lingerie and studied out-of-print books on the subject (all the more reason that we are so lucky today to hold Cora's wisdom within these pages!). So when I first started performing striptease, I distinguished myself from the other dancers in their contemporary underwear by hooking into (and out of) corsets and seamed stockings. It was a daring business decision in 1992. But I loved the way these old-fashioned wares made me feel. I could create the kind of mythic fantasy I long admired on the screen. I felt beautiful in them.

A wonderful career as a burlesque performer, a few lingerie-clad cameos on the runways, and too many photo shoots to count have followed those days. Today, I get some of the greatest pleasure designing lingerie—with all those in mind whom I've met and performed for over the years. For them—for you—I strive to make bewitching, well-fitting lingerie that is accessible in price and in sizing. We all think we have flaws, and I believe in distracting from those flaws, imagined or real, by accentuating the positive. I get such joy seeing individuals of different body shapes and sizes and skin tones embrace lingerie as a way to celebrate themselves.

Which begs the fundamental question of them all: Why would anyone not want to wear lingerie?

Dita Von Teese

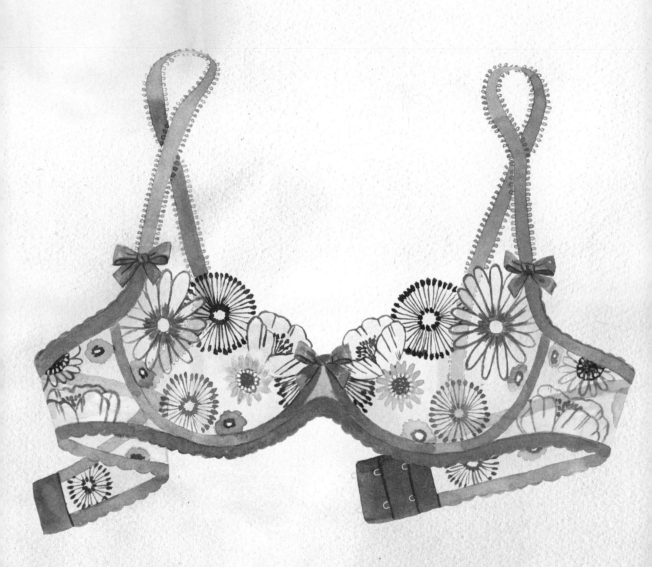

Introduction

L et's be honest: lingerie is confusing. There are thousands of brands, hundreds of styles, and dozens of sizes. Even if you like the *idea* of lingerie, intimate apparel can be a complicated and bewildering world. What's the difference between a demi bra and a balconette? What's the point of having seams on a bra? More important, how do you find the right bra for you? Moving beyond bras, what kind of lingerie should you wear for formal occasions, your honeymoon, or even a regular workday? This book answers all that and more.

Why Lingerie?

Often, when I tell people that I write about lingerie, their first question is, "What's the point?" And that's understandable. Lingerie is mysterious. Most of us wear it in some form or another every day, but we don't know much about it. What can good, functional, high-quality, and beautiful lingerie add to your life? Why should you pay special attention to your underthings at all? What if you're plus-size or older or have never spent more than five minutes in the lingerie section of a department store?

For many of us, lingerie can feel like a fancy party we weren't invited to. All those delicate pieces might look pretty in a shop window or online but once you have them in hand and try them on, it can feel as though lingerie wasn't made with you in mind at all. Does that mean lingerie is useless? Is it only for the supermodels among us?

No. Not at all.

Nice lingerie is for everyone. It's for you. It's for me. It's for anyone who wants it. This book breaks down the barriers around lingerie, answers questions, simplifies hard-to-understand concepts, and makes sense of all the little things the experts take for granted. My hope is that by the end of this book, the world of lingerie will feel more accessible, more understandable, and, above all, like something you can continue to explore on your own. The emphasis here is on practical knowledge you can apply throughout your life for years to come—not on trends or fads.

While lingerie can be baffling, puzzling, and sometimes even outright frightening, the good news is there's never been a better time to become interested in lingerie. The number of sizes, brands, price points, and styles available at this moment in lingerie history is completely unparalleled. No matter your interest, aim, or situation, there is someone, somewhere, making lingerie with you in mind—for your body, your style, your taste, and your budget. *In Intimate Detail* is about giving you the tools you need to discover and confidently wear and care for these pieces.

In this book, you'll find recommendations for a range of body types, physical conditions, and life events. Why? Because our bodies are wonderful and glorious and amazing, and we all deserve to wear beautiful lingerie.

However, there is one thing this book is *not* about, and that's giving you rules about what you *should* wear. While you may see notes to give you fit advice or tell you about a certain style, I want you to use the information in *In Intimate Detail* as you see fit. There is no single way to wear lingerie. You should wear what you love and what makes you feel good, because you deserve that.

Throughout this book, you'll learn things like how to choose lingerie for your particular breast shape and fashion preferences, how to recognize high-quality lingerie, how to interpret industry terms (such as the difference between *full bust* and *plus size*), how to take care of your lingerie, and even how to give it as a gift. *In Intimate Detail* covers more specialty topics too, such as bra advice for those expecting a child and how to buy underwear if you're coping with menopause. While I won't claim this book covers *everything*—I know that's impossible—I've tried to make this book the kind of resource that I wish had existed when I first became interested in lingerie.

You'll find advice and information on different types of intimate apparel—such as bras, underwear, shapewear, hosiery, and loungewear—followed by sections on how to apply your newfound practical knowledge when shopping for lingerie (both online and in boutiques or department stores), as well as how to care for it. Feel free to skip around and pick and choose which bits you'd like to read first.

There's another reason you should be a more informed and more knowledgeable lingerie buyer: you can demand better from the lingerie industry and from the brands that are making these products for you. An informed consumer is a powerful consumer. When you know what's *available* as well as what's *possible*, you can ask for better from the brands that make your underwear. Customer demand is the number-one incentive for brands to change things, and this book will give you the tools and the vocabulary you need to help make the changes you want to see happen.

I've always believed lingerie is fashion too—that what we wear underneath is just as important as what's worn on top. When talking about fashion or how to shop or what to wear, lingerie is often overlooked, but it's as much a part of a stylish wardrobe as the perfect handbag, classic blazer, or chic little black dress. More than that, good lingerie helps us feel better about our bodies and ourselves. And it can help our clothes fit better too!

By the end of this book, you'll have an expert's perspective on all the major highlights of the lingerie world. You'll know what lingerie is right for you and why. You'll have a better understanding of how and where to buy it and some little tricks and shortcuts for building your own uniquely beautiful lingerie collection. You'll also find several appendices at the end of this book with a few practical lists, including an international bra size conversion chart. Finally, the appendices are also where you'll find information for special concerns, such as lingerie advice for those transitioning, living with fibromyalgia, or coping with the aftereffects of a mastectomy. But first, let's make sure we're on the same page about what lingerie actually is.

What Is Lingerie?

Lingerie serves many purposes. It warms the body, protects our outer garments, offers modesty, and provides a barrier between our skin and harsh fabrics. Lingerie also supports the body and helps shape the figure according to current standards of beauty. Christian Dior once said, "Without foundations, there can be no fashion." Fashion depends on lingerie. In the seventeenth century, a conically shaped torso was *en vogue*. A couple of centuries later, an hourglass figure was all the rage. A hundred years after that, fashion couldn't get enough of the "natural" look. In every era, lingerie changes to support or even create the fashionable figure of the day.

However, lingerie is also a physical representation of our culture. Intimate apparel embodies a number of codes or rules—things that are usually unspoken but taken for granted. More than perhaps any other category of fashion, lingerie is full of significance and meaning. Maybe that's why society gives us mixed messages regarding what our lingerie should be. We're told that lingerie is required for us to dress "appropriately," but also that it's frivolous, pointless, and foolish.

However, I believe lingerie is more than practical scaffolding for your outerwear. It's also a way to care for, treat, and pamper yourself. Unlike all the other things you may need to wear to make others happy, lingerie can truly be about dressing for yourself. Lingerie isn't intimate apparel just because it's hidden; it's intimate because it can reflect your innermost self, your secret identity. That's powerful.

The word *lingerie* comes from the French word *linge*, or linen. Chemises, which were an essential part of a woman's wardrobe from the Middle Ages until about the nineteenth century, were made from linen, a strong, comfortable fabric that could withstand the harsh laundry soaps of the day. Most dresses, especially those worn by the wealthy, could not be submerged in water, and poorer people wouldn't necessarily have the time or changes of clothes necessary to wash their outer garments more frequently. Therefore, these chemises were worn directly against the skin and helped to protect more expensive outerwear from the sweat and grime of unwashed skin. By the nineteenth century, the word *lingerie* was used to refer to undergarments, specifically loosely fitting items like chemises and drawers. All other undergarments—especially shaping undergarments like corsets, bras, and girdles—were referred to as *corsetry*.

While many people think of lingerie as only the sexy stuff—bedroom attire, so to speak—lingerie is a category of women's fashion, not something limited to a specific activity. Lingerie includes all women's underwear, sleepwear, loungewear, and shapewear. Recent trends like athleisure and lingerie-as-outerwear have blurred the lines between intimate apparel and "regular" fashion. Generally speaking, if it's meant to be worn under your clothing, worn exclusively at home, or worn to bed, it's probably lingerie. That means lingerie isn't just bras and panties; it's also slips, chemises, shapewear, pajamas, robes, stockings, tights, nightgowns, and teddies. Lingerie includes the expensive, special-occasion stuff and the everyday, basic stuff. *It's all lingerie.*

Just like our outerwear, our underwear can be a form of self-expression. In the same way your jewelry, makeup, shoes, coat, and handbag reflect your personality and tastes, so too can your lingerie. No matter what you show to the rest of world, your lingerie can be the truest expression of who you are. It can be something worn just for you because you want to, and that can be incredibly empowering. It can even be life changing.

While many people equate lingerie with sex and sexuality, lingerie does not always have to be erotic wear. And while intimate apparel often serves a practical purpose, such as helping clothes fit better, it shouldn't just be about changing or "fixing" the body. And lingerie should *never* be painful to wear or a source of shame.

Lingerie is about self-expression, identity, art, and joy. It's about fun, playfulness, and experimentation. Feeling like a silver-screen siren? Swan about the house in a long satin robe. Looking for a quick boost of confidence? Wear your favorite black bra and panty set underneath your regular clothes. Ready to start a new exercise regimen? Splurge on that funky, brightly colored sports bra. Your lingerie wardrobe doesn't have to be limited to what's boring or "practical." It can be whatever you want. That's the beauty of lingerie.

BONUS TIP

The best lingerie sales happen in January and July.

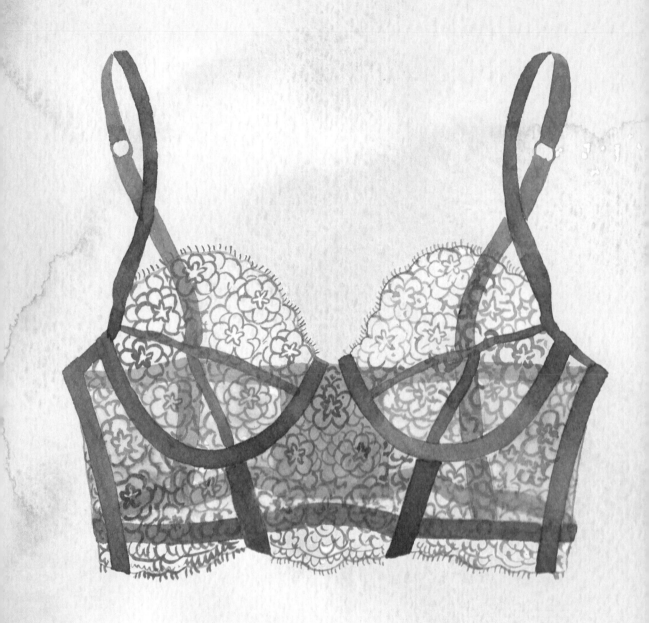

CHAPTER 1

_____

BRAS

A great, well-fitting bra can help you feel confident, empowered, and fearless. Finding the right bra can almost feel like stumbling across your very own version of Cinderella's magic slippers, transforming your life (and your wardrobe!) from depressing to enchanting. A good bra can not only lift your bust, it can lift your spirits—alleviating back pain, evenly distributing the weight of your breasts, and even improving your posture.

Because most clothing is made with certain assumptions about where the largest area of your chest will be, a quality bra can also help your clothes fit better and feel more comfortable. Finally, bras can be fun! I know that might be hard to believe if you've had trouble shopping for a bra, but a new bra is a great way to both treat yourself and refresh your wardrobe.

A Brief History of Bras

Interestingly enough, no one's really sure who made the first bra. In the United States, the story goes that Caresse Crosby (also known as Mary Phelps Jacob) invented the first brassiere around 1910 when she wanted an alternative to the traditional boned corset. Together with her maid, Crosby crafted a bra from two handkerchiefs and a bit of ribbon, filed a patent, and in February 1914, the bra was officially recognized and registered in the United States. Crosby's invention was more like a bralette (a bra with little or no structure) than the kind of undergarments we call bras today. However, what made her bra special is that it was soft, flexible, lightweight, and comfortable—a dramatic change from centuries of rigid corsets. However, despite filing a patent and being credited with the invention, it's almost certainly true that Caresse Crosby's bra was not the first one *ever*.

The first bras of prehistory were likely made from strips of hide or fur to bind the breasts. Later, after its invention, cloth was also used. Four-thousand-year-old paintings and sculptures from Crete show female figures with their breasts lifted from beneath by a corset-like garment. Greek sculptures from the fourth century BCE, display women in breast bands consisting of a wide strip of cloth wound around the breasts to keep them in place.

WHAT IS A BRA?

A bra is a garment designed and developed specifically to support the breasts. A bra may extend as far as the lower torso (as in longline bras or bustiers). However, undergarments that sculpt and shape other parts of the body in addition to the bosom (such as shaping slips or bodysuits) are rarely called bras. A bra, by definition, focuses primarily on the bust.

Paintings and mosaics from the time of the Roman Empire present women in two-piece undergarment sets that look strikingly like a modern-day bra and briefs. We've even found a bra dating from the late Middle Ages, roughly around the fifteenth century! Made of linen, featuring two distinct cups, and trimmed in delicate needlepoint lace, this garment is the earliest physical example of a bra found yet (although they were called *breast bags* at the time, a decidedly unglamorous name).

The modern bra, as a concept, has its origins in corsetry (so does shapewear, which you'll learn more about in chapter 3). The idea of supporting and shaping the body beneath clothing came into vogue around the invention of tailoring, which roughly coincides with the beginnings of the Renaissance, around the fourteenth century. The figure-hugging, tightly laced dresses of the Middle Ages gradually gave way to the firmly boned bodices, known as *stays*, of the sixteenth century.

Stays gave the body a cone-like shape. Heavily boned, their purpose in addition to supporting and lifting the bust was to brace the body for the pounds and pounds of heavy skirts women were beginning to wear. Stays remained the bust-supporting undergarment *de rigueur* for women until the French Revolution.

The French were among the first to see corsetry as necessary for a woman's figure, and their attitude regarding underpinnings spread to other European courts. However, after the French Revolution, both stays and the massive volumes of skirts they helped support were seen as suspiciously aristocratic. At the end of the eighteenth century, a more natural empire-waist silhouette emerged. These soft, fluid gowns called for a different type of undergarment, which led to the development of the first "proto-bras." Called *short stays*, these abbreviated corsets ended above the waist and featured separate cups, resembling what we might call a *bustier* today.

However, this new trend didn't last long, and thirty years into the nineteenth century, the corset made a comeback, this time emphasizing an hourglass figure instead of a conical one. The development of steel busks and metal eyelets allowed for a drawn-in waist and lifted bust. Yet the short stays of the early 1800s had left their mark, and in the late nineteenth century, a plethora of new "brassiere" designs emerged. While these early bras don't have much in common appearance-wise with what we wear today, the concepts were there: bust support, separate cups for each breast, adjustable shoulder straps, and even hook-and-eye closures.

So what finally killed the corset? Well, sports played a part. Women began to participate in tennis, golf, basketball, swimming, and cycling—all activities for which the corset has obvious limitations. Yet it wasn't the bicycle that wiped out the corset for good. Instead, we can pin its final demise on World War I.

In 1917, just three years after Caresse Crosby received her patent, the U.S. War Industries Board asked women to stop buying corsets so the steel "bones" could be freed up for the war. Their sacrifice made more than twenty-eight thousand tons of steel available—enough to build two battleships. Meanwhile, as women gave up their corsets, they also went to work in munitions factories, fire departments, and other occupations previously closed to them. As with athletics, the shortcomings (and potential dangers) of the corset, with its many bones and laces, became apparent. By 1918, more than fifty-two separate bra brands were on the market. The shift away from corsetry was complete.

By the 1920s, most corset makers had fully converted to making bras or the new, more modern girdles. In the 1930s, cup sizes, elastic, and underwires became a regular feature of the bra landscape. The word *bra* also first appeared in the 1930s. While the fashionable bra silhouette of the 1920s favored a bandeau style, which offered little support and mostly worked to flatten the bust, in the 1930s, the idea of the bra as a lifting and separating device took shape. By the 1940s, almost all Western women were wearing bras, and, as the saying goes, the rest is history.

A very high, perky bust was the trademark of the 1950s (bullet bras, with their world-famous torpedo cups, dominated the lingerie landscape in this era). The 1960s and 1970s favored a softer, more natural silhouette. Bras of this era were often sheer and lightweight, incorporating radical new stretch fabrics, which emphasized mobility and flexibility. The sports bra was also invented in the 1970s.

The 1980s saw a return of more structured bras, as well as a rise in the concept of the "invisible" bra—bras with smooth or lightly seamed cups that were intended not to be seen under clothing. The 1990s brought an obsession with deep plunges and push-up padding. Now, instead of simply shaping what you had, bras could add several cup sizes all on their own. In the 2000s, seamless, one-piece molded- and foam-cup bras became ubiquitous, replacing the cut-and-sew styles of previous generations and leading to that familiar dome or half-moon shape we all recognize today. More recently, the natural silhouette has made a comeback in the form of the bralette, but fashion is cyclical, and who knows when one of the bra trends of yesteryear will experience a revival?

The Parts of a Bra

Bras may look simple but they are actually highly specialized and very complex articles of clothing. The average bra contains dozens of components, and each, no matter how small, has a specific purpose. All these pieces must be put together by hand, so the time involved in sewing a bra is a large part of why bras are so expensive, despite their small size.

Understanding the construction of a bra can help you better describe what you like or dislike about a particular style or shape, and it can help you discover which kind of bra is best for you.

Cups

The cups of the bra are where your breasts sit. Usually rounded, as that's the current fashion (think of your favorite T-shirt or contour cup bra), the cups section can also be pointed (as in a bullet bra) or even slightly collapsed (as in a seamed bra that won't fill out until it's on the body). In most bras, this area consists of two distinct cups, but certain bra styles, such as bandeaus or sports bras, have a single cup section meant to contain both breasts. Cups may be lined or unlined, as well as seamed or seamless. The underwires of your bra, if it has them, are also cup components, usually running in special channels along the bottom and sides of the cups.

Band

The most important part of the bra, the band is responsible for providing most of the support. The band handles up to 80 percent of the work of supporting your breasts (which means your straps shouldn't be doing much at all!) and includes everything that wraps around the torso. The band can be broken down into four distinct parts: the *center panel*—otherwise known as the gore or bridge—which connects the two cups together in the middle; the *cradle*, which is the portion of the band directly underneath the cups or underwires (not present in "bandless" bra styles); the *wings*, which are the sides and back of the bra, starting at the outer edge of the cups and ending at the closures; and the closures, usually consisting of hooks and eyes, but sometimes made of other materials. Note: If you're wearing a front-close bra, the center panel and the closure are the same.

Straps

Straps help keep your bra stable and in place. They go over your shoulders (excepting, of course, strapless and halter bra styles) but are not meant to support the entire weight of your breasts. They should account for about 20 percent of the lift. The area where the straps meet the cups is called the *apex*. Straps are almost always adjustable, even in the most basic of bra styles. There are two popular types of strap attachments: the camisole (otherwise known as a right-angle or straight-back attachment) and a leotard (otherwise known as a ballet back or u-back attachment). The latter tends to be better for fuller busts (DD cups and above), as well as for narrower shoulders, as the straps are less likely to slide or fall.

Underwires

We've all seen an underwire bra before, but exactly what purpose does that little piece of curved wire at the bottom of your bra cup serve? Basically, why do bras have underwires?

Underwires have been around since 1931, and contrary to a popular rumor, the invention of the underwire is attributed to a woman—Helene Pons. It was another couple of decades before

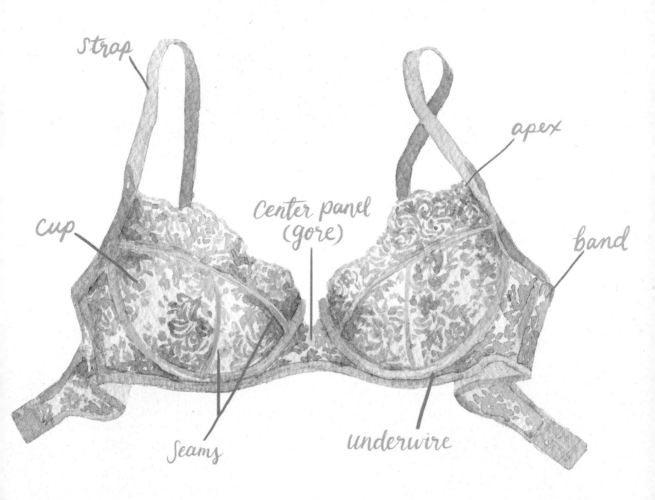

strap

apex

cup

center panel
(gore)

band

Seams

underwire

underwire bras overtook wireless styles in popularity. As with the corset, a war (World War II) needed to end before enough metal was available to explore the possibilities of the underwire.

An underwire is essentially an idealized *breast root*—the curve on the body where the breast tissue attaches to the torso. Underwires are meant to follow the contour of the breast, providing shaping and support from the bottom of the bra (the cradle and band area).

An underwire is usually narrower than the breast itself, which helps contain the breast tissue (it helps "scoop" it all into the cup). In conjunction with the bra cups, the underwire tells your breasts what shape to take and which direction to go, and this is what gives them an uplifted silhouette.

Underwires are typically made of metal, though occasionally they can be made of plastic or silicone. Bras for larger bust sizes, such as those over a DD cup, tend to contain sturdier wires to accommodate the weight of a heavier breast. Assuming there's no underlying pain or condition, such as fibromyalgia, underwires shouldn't hurt. So if a wire is bruising you, digging in, or otherwise feeling uncomfortable, it may be the wrong shape for your particular breast root, or it is too aggressive for your breast tissue. As always, listen to your body. If it doesn't feel good, don't wear it.

Seams

Bra seams offer more than decoration. They're essential for shaping the bust. In the United States, seamless contour cup bras are the most popular. However, a contour cup is not the most supportive type of bra, especially for large busts. That's not a flaw; it's simply a side effect of the limits of molded-cup technology.

The molded cup works by forcing your breast into a certain position. The bra doesn't change its shape to accommodate your bust. Your bust changes shape to fit into the bra. That means whatever shape the molded cup has is the shape your breasts will have.

Unfortunately, how effective that shape is depends on the resilience of the fabrics and materials making up the cup. Beyond a certain size, a molded cup simply can't adequately support the weight of a heavier bust. Even if you can technically wear the bra, it won't be able to shape the tissue as well as it could for a smaller bust. That's why bra brands that focus on larger sizes offer more seamed or cut-and-sew-style bras. It's also why almost all bras beyond an H cup are cut-and-sew.

Seams gently guide the breast tissue into a specific shape. Keep in mind that the more seams a bra has, the more supportive it will be.

- **Vertical seams:** These seams direct the breast tissue upward, providing lift. The more vertical seams a bra has, the more lift and support you'll get.

- **Horizontal seams:** These seams help give more forward depth to the cups, also known as *projection*. Sometimes, however, this seam can lead to what people call a "pointy silhouette."

- **Diagonal or angled seams:** These seams help center the breast tissue, pulling it away from the shoulders and armpits, and also provide lift. You'll often see a diagonal seam used in conjunction with a vertical seam for the classic three-part cup shape (this is the cup shape shown in the diagram on page 13). Together, these seams lift, center, and shape the breast tissue.

- **Side seams or side panels:** These seams run from the top to the bottom of the cup, usually along the outer edge. They are something extra that you'll find in full-bust and plus-sized bras. The side panel helps make sure all the breast tissue is pulled away from the sides of the body and contained within the bra cups, front and center. For people with larger breasts, side seams help create a smaller profile.

Bra seams aren't something to be intimidated by—they're just a tool. Seams not only improve your bra's fit, but also reinforce the cup structure. And if you're a fan of beautiful bras, here's some good news: cut-and-sew bras tend to use much prettier fabrics than contour cup bras. If you've tried all the contour cup bras available and found that none of them work for you, give seams a try. You may be surprised!

Why Wear a Bra?

I'm not here to give you lingerie rules, but I do want to give you as much information as I can. There are lots of good reasons to wear a bra. As I mentioned, bras can help with back, shoulder, and neck pain. They can improve posture, help keep the breasts from bouncing (which can be especially painful during physical activity), and provide a layer of protection or insulation between sensitive parts of the body, such as the nipples, and your outerwear. Bras can also help support confidence. Not having to think about your breasts and their comfort during the day means you can focus on other, more important things. And, of course, since most of our clothing is made with the assumption that we will be wearing a bra, bras can help our garments fit better on our bodies.

However, there is one thing bras do not prevent, and that's breast sagging (ptosis). I know . . . I'm probably turning everything you've heard about this on its head, but stay with me because this is important. According to medical research, there are five major causes of ptosis, and none of them involve wearing a bra: smoking, significant weight loss and/or gain, pregnancy (*not* breastfeeding), growing older, and just plain-old genetics (which also determines the softness of your breast tissue, the elasticity of your skin, and the size and shape of your breasts, in general).

I can't tell you how many people have come to me nearly in tears, worried they've "ruined" their breasts due to not wearing a bra or because they have been wearing a poorly fitting bra. Please know that no matter how your breasts look, they are not "ruined." And you, as a human being, are certainly not "ruined." You are more than your breasts.

It may seem strange to include a section in a chapter about bras telling you that bras won't permanently change your breasts or ultimately make your breasts look any different than they do now, but I believe it's important for people to have accurate information so they can make informed decisions . . . instead of relying on fear, rumors, or myths.

If you enjoy wearing a bra, keep wearing a bra. And if you feel like you need to wear a bra, *for whatever reason*, then you should wear a bra. I'm not here to tell you to stop or start doing anything. But please don't think you're doing bras "wrong" if your breasts don't look like that perky model's in the fashion magazine. More than likely, whether because of Photoshop trickery or just plain genetics, that model's appearance is due to factors completely beyond your control.

Bra Sizes

A bra size—whether it's 32A, 38C, 34DD, 28J, or 42K—is really just a ratio. The number, or band size, roughly corresponds to the size of your rib cage or underbust. The letter, or cup size, represents the difference between your rib cage and your bust at its fullest point.

To get the letter, use a cloth tape measure to take your bust and then your underbust measurements. Subtract the second number from the first one. Every inch of difference corresponds to one cup size. For example, if your bust measurement is forty inches and your underbust measurement is thirty-six inches, your bra size would be, approximately, 36D (thirty-six inches being your rib-cage measurement, and the D cup reflecting the four inches of difference between that measurement and your bust at its fullest point).

One inch of difference is an A cup, two inches of difference is a B cup, three inches of difference is a C cup, and four inches of difference is a D cup. Five inches, though? Well, here's where a pesky lack of standardization comes in: U.S. bra manufacturers rarely venture beyond the letter D for cup size; instead they repeat it (D, DD, DDD, DDDD, and so on). U.K. bra companies use single letters, then double, then single again, starting with the D cup (D, DD, E, F, FF, and so on). And European bra brands progress straight through the alphabet (A to H). So for U.S. and U.K. brands, a five-inch difference is a DD, but for European brands, it's an E.

Fortunately, you don't have to remember all of this: when trying new brands, reference both the brand's in-house size chart as well as the International Bra Cup Size Conversion Chart on page 137, where you'll find comparisons of U.S., U.K., and European sizes.

Here's where things get even more tricky, though, because there are two major schools of thought when it comes to finding your

BRA SIZING SCHOOLS OF THOUGHT

The Classic Method: Add four or five inches to your underbust measurement to arrive at your bra band size (it's "four or five" because there are no odd-numbered band sizes for bras, so you'll need to add five inches if your rib cage is an odd number). To put this into practice, if your rib cage is thirty inches around, your bra band would be a size 34. Using this method doesn't mean the band is thirty-four inches long; it's still cut for a thirty-inch rib cage. The only thing that has changed is the final number, much like how a size-16 dress doesn't correspond to sixteen inches of anything; it's just a number on the tag.

The New Method: Your underbust measurement corresponds exactly to your band-size number. So a thirty-inch underbust equals a thirty-inch band size (this is the example given in "Bra Sizes" on this page).

bra size: the Classic Method and the New Method (also known as the Plus Four and the Plus Zero methods, respectively; see "Bra Sizing Schools of Thought" on page 17). The style you use will depend on the bra brand you wear. There is very little consistency in the lingerie industry, partly because every bra company chooses the sizing method they prefer. While it is confusing to learn both, having them in mind will help you be a better bra shopper and find the bras that work best for you.

Very generally speaking, bra brands for DD and above cups will use the New Method (that is, your exact underbust measurement for your band size), while bra brands specializing in A to D cups will use the Classic Method. You'll know which method the brand uses if you check the fitting or sizing section on the company website or if you ask the salesperson in a bra boutique or department store. While it may seem unnecessary to know both, it's important to remember that bra sizes aren't static, and the size you wear often depends on the brand. This is why it's entirely normal to have two or three different sizes in your bra drawer and for them all to fit perfectly.

The most important takeaway I want you to have from this section is that, no matter what bra size you wear and no matter what sizing system you use, *all* bra sizes are normal and okay. Even if you've been frustrated before, there's a good chance someone, somewhere is making the bra of your dreams—and being aware of all this information about sizing can help you find it.

Sister Sizes

As you now know, your bra size is essentially shorthand for two separate measurements: your overbust and your underbust. Said another way, your bra size is a rough estimation of your breast volume, that is, the amount of space your breasts would occupy if they weren't attached to your body.

A *sister size* is when the band and cup size of your bra changes but the *cup volume* (the amount of breast tissue the bra can hold) remains the same. Because sister sizing gives you more bra options to choose from, knowing this can be helpful if you wear

PLUS SIZE VERSUS FULL BUST

As you've likely noticed, the lingerie world has a lot of unique terminology. When you're bra shopping, keep in mind the difference between *plus size* and *full bust*. Many brands use those terms interchangeably, but they mean two very different things, and understanding that difference can help make bra shopping much easier.

Plus size usually refers to a band size of 38 or above. Although some plus-sized bra manufacturers make band sizes as small as 34 or 36 (because a rib-cage measurement of thirty-six inches is very different on someone who's five feet tall versus six feet tall), most bra retailers won't refer to a bra size as plus size until it passes that 38–40 band mark. If you're plus-sized, you want to buy from retailers who specialize in that size range, because those brands really know their stuff about plus-sized bodies. They're specialists and experts, and they will make the best-fitting and highest-quality bras for your size.

Full bust refers to a cup size of DD or above. That DD cup mark is usually the point at which a bra's pattern and style must change to accommodate the needs of a larger, heavier bust. That point is called a size break, and there is another size break around the H cup mark. While it can be frustrating to have to buy bras from specialty brands when you have a fuller bust, they are worth investing in because those companies use fabrics, wires, patterns, and finishes specifically designed to make the very best and most supportive bras for larger cup sizes. Don't set yourself up for disappointment. Go to the experts for your size first.

BRALESS OPTIONS

Not everyone wears a bra, for various and personal reasons. Sometimes medical concerns, allergies, or skin sensitivity mean wearing a bra simply isn't an option. Other times, it's a matter of personal preference, identity, or self-expression. Whatever your reason, there are a lot of bra-free options available now that are worth knowing about.

Adhesive nipple covers, silicone pasties, breast tape, bodysuits, camisoles, and other garments with built-in bust seaming or darting can help replace a bra. These items also provide layers, which can disguise the outline of a nipple or an unsupported breast silhouette. Speaking of layers, thicker layers (such as sweaters and sweatshirts) can be useful as well, but even several thin layers (such as a crop top over a leotard) can provide a similar blurring effect.

a hard-to-find size or have special fit concerns, such as a flared rib cage or skin sensitivity.

To find your sister size, go up a band size and down a cup size if you're looking for a larger band, or up a cup size and down a band size if you prefer a smaller band. For example, this is the lineup of sister sizes that go with my bra size (34C): 38A, 36B, 32D, and 30DD.

Knowing your sister size is useful for accommodating size and weight fluctuations. Your sister size is also helpful if bras in your "real size" are difficult to shop for, but bras in your sister size are more common (or less expensive) to buy. In particular, people with smaller rib cages and proportionately larger busts or people with larger rib cages and proportionately smaller busts will benefit most from sister sizing.

Generally speaking, you won't want to sister size out more than two sizes in either direction. Beyond that, significant changes to the bra pattern mean you likely won't get a good fit. For example, bras in cup sizes DD and above tend to use firmer materials and narrower underwires than A to D cup sizes; these added features are usually more supportive and more comfortable for a heavier bust. If your measured bra size is an H cup but you sister size into a D cup, there's a good possibility you won't get the shaping and support you might want from your bras.

One incredibly important thing sister sizing reveals is that cup size isn't static across band sizes. Said another way, there is no such thing as a DD cup all on its own: 28DD, 32DD, 38DD, 44DD, and 50DD all have very different cup volumes. They're each made for a completely different bra size. This is why lingerie experts will want to know your band size in addition to your cup size—DD simply doesn't convey enough information.

No matter what the numbers and letters on the tag say, what matters most is finding the bra size that works for *you*. That might mean changing the size you've worn for years. It might even mean that you wear a different bra size than your friend or family member who has the exact same measurements. And it'll probably mean that you have two or three different sizes in your lingerie drawer. That's all normal. Please don't suffer in an uncomfortable, ill-fitting bra. Cut out the tags if you have to, but wear a bra that makes you feel good . . . not one that makes you feel miserable.

Breast Shape

Knowing your breast shape is just as important as knowing your bra size when it comes to lingerie shopping. All breast shapes are normal, but being able to identify your particular breast shape can help you find the bras that will work best for you.

Before we go any further, I want to address breast unevenness or asymmetry. I get so many questions from people who wonder if having one breast larger than the other is normal or if there's something wrong with them. Here's the thing: *everyone*, unless they've undergone breast augmentation or reconstructive surgery, has differently sized breasts. Usually, the left breast is larger than the right. Differences between the two breasts can range from very slight and barely noticeable to a cup size or more. If there is a significant size difference between your breasts, you want to fit your bra to the larger breast and use a *cookie*, or insert, to fill out the cup for the smaller breast. And while consistent breast-size differences are normal, if you notice a sudden, abrupt change in size or shape, please see a doctor.

While there are as many breast shapes and types as there are people, the following five breast shapes will have the most impact on your bra-fitting experience.

Full on Bottom

Full-on-bottom breasts mean most of your breast mass or weight is located on the lower half of the breast, beneath the nipple line. Plunge styles are especially good for full-on-bottom shapes, as are demi cups.

Full on Top

Full-on-top breasts mean most of your breast volume is located within the upper half of the breast, usually above the nipple line. Balcony bras and other styles that are open at the top of the cup

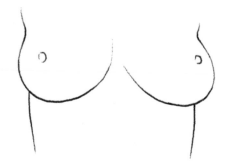

FULL ON BOTTOM

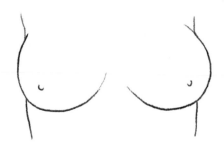

FULL ON TOP

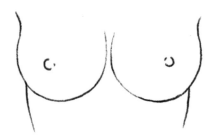

FULL ALL AROUND

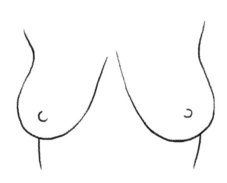

PENDULOUS

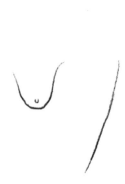

TUBEROUS

are perfect for full-on-top shapes. Full-coverage bras with a stretchy lace upper panel are also a good fit.

Full All Around

Full-all-around breasts have evenly distributed fullness around the top and bottom halves of the breast (that is, you have roughly equal amounts of breast tissue above and below the nipple). Full-all-around breasts often appear round or spherical, and this is often the shape of the breast after augmentation surgery (though, obviously, not all full-all-around breasts are augmented). Most bra styles work well for full-all-around shapes, including balconette, full-coverage, and plunge styles.

Pendulous

Pendulous breasts are softer breasts where most of the breast tissue hangs below the breast root (where your breast attaches to your body). Your breast shape can be full on bottom or full on top in addition to pendulous, because those first two definitions hinge primarily on nipple placement; however, pendulous breasts usually lack volume. Pendulous breasts are common in all ages; wearing or not wearing a bra has nothing to do with having a pendulous shape. That said, sometimes breasts can become more pendulous after pregnancy or with age. Full-coverage bras and bras with cut-and-sew cups will help shape the breast, giving it lift and projection.

Tuberous

Tuberous (also known as tubular) breasts have very little breast tissue and are characterized by an elongated, narrow, and cylindrical shape—like a tube. Other characteristics of tuberous breasts include large, puffy areolas, wide spacing between them, and a narrow breast root. Molded or padded push-up or plunge styles (such as T-shirt bras) help give tuberous breasts a more even and projected shape.

In addition to knowing your breast shape, it's useful to be able to identify if your breasts are widely or narrowly spaced.

Narrowly Spaced

Narrowly spaced or close-set breasts mean your breasts are very close together and may even touch at the top of your chest. If you find that the center panel of your bra rarely rests flat against your sternum but is instead sitting on top of breast tissue, you may have closely set breasts. Bras with low, short, and narrow center panels (as in many demi and plunge styles), work well and are most comfortable for narrowly spaced breasts.

Widely Spaced

Widely spaced breasts are farther apart on the chest, usually wider than two or three finger widths apart. Interestingly, plunge bras can also work well for this breast placement! Widely spaced breasts often cannot achieve that pushed-together cleavage look, but Marie Antoinette–style cleavage (of the "heaving bosoms" variety) is still an option with widely spaced breasts. Front-closure styles and balconette bras are also good for this breast placement.

Shallow/Projected

Finally, it's good to know if your breasts are shallow or projected. It's best to think of shallowness and projection on a spectrum (as opposed to two entirely separate and distinct characteristics) describing how much space on your chest your breasts occupy.

Shallower breasts tend to have a broad base and occupy much of the width of the chest laterally, but they don't project very far away from the chest wall. Projected breasts cover less of the chest wall (that is, they have a narrower root or point of attachment to the chest) but stick out farther from the body. To use an analogy, the concept of shallow versus projected is a bit like putting liquid into a plate versus a bowl. Even if you pour the same amount of liquid, it will take up a *wider* amount of space in the plate but a *higher* amount of space in the bowl. Shallow breasts are usually full on bottom as well (and may even appear "pointy," especially from the side), while projected breasts may be full on bottom, full on top, or full all around.

Demi, balconette, and plunge styles, especially those with open tops and wide wires, are perfect for shallower shapes as there's not usually enough projected breast tissue to fill out a full-coverage cup. Deep bra cups with narrow wires are ideally suited to projected shapes and may be found in plunge, balconette, or full-coverage styles.

As always, these are just general guidelines and suggestions. Nothing—not me, not this book, not anyone—can replace trying on bras for yourself and discovering what you love best.

Types of Bras

Now that you know your size and your breast shape, it's time to talk bra styles. Following are twenty-four of the most popular types of bras. Keep in mind that a single bra can cross two or even three categories on this list (for example: a strapless, cut-and-sew longline or a plunge, wireless, maternity bra). In addition, as with everything else in the lingerie industry, not all brands are in agreement on which terms should be used for which bras. Think of these groups as broad, general categories to help you use the right language when bra shopping.

Adhesive

Adhesive bras are usually strapless and backless, and they stay on the body with medical-grade adhesive or sticky tape, sometimes in combination with silicone for traction and "grip" (hence their other name, *stick-on bra*). Adhesive bras are the ultimate wardrobe solution, offering coverage and shape for even the most revealing garments, such as backless, strapless, and deep-plunge styles. Their biggest downside? They're not supportive and give very little lift, a potential deal breaker for heavier busts.

Balconette

A balconette (or balcony) bra is a type of half-cup bra and is essentially a lower-cut or less-coverage demi style with prominent vertical seams. Balconette bras have wide necklines, and, in their most dramatic variation, the top of each cup is cut straight across, giving a profile reminiscent of a balcony—hence the name. In addition to wide necklines, balconette bras tend to have widely spaced straps, making them a potentially difficult fit for people

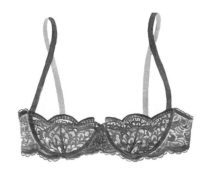

with narrow shoulders (the straps can slide off too easily). Balconette bras give high, rounded cleavage and are a go-to style for those with broad shoulders and full-on-bottom breasts. For everyday wear, balconette styles are ideally suited for low-cut tops. As a sidenote, some readers, especially those who wear DD cup sizes or higher, may find that balconettes in their size range more closely resemble demi cups, and vice versa!

Bandeau

A version of the bandeau has been worn since ancient times, making this the original bra. Nowadays, bandeaus are made from a wide band of stretchy fabric. Usually lacking closures or underwires, bandeaus resemble a shortened tube top and are essentially a less-structured version of a strapless bra. Because of their lack of structure, bandeaus offer very little support or shaping, which can make them a difficult fit for larger breasts but a fun and easy wardrobe option for smaller busts. Bandeaus are typically available in a wide range of colors, prints, and laces, which make them perfect for peeking out from under a tank top or maxi dress.

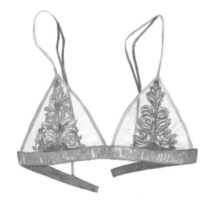

Bralette

Like the bandeau, a bralette is an unstructured or lightly structured bra without wires and with few seams. Bralettes may be lined or unlined. They may have either front or rear closures or can be slipped on over the head. Many bralettes resemble a triangle bikini top or a crop top. The bra Mary Phelps Jacob invented in the early twentieth century would likely have been called a bralette today. Bralettes are a comfortable, laid-back, no-fuss option, and, like bandeaus, are also popular among people with smaller busts (though anyone can wear them). However, they are not supportive and do little to shape or lift the breasts. Some people like to wear bralettes as sleep or lounge bras at home, especially when the bralette is made from a soft, comfortable fiber like bamboo or cotton. (See page 50 for more information on fiber types.)

Bullet

A vintage style, bullet bras were popular in the 1950s and famous for their concentric circles of stitching around the bra cup. This stitching created a pointed bullet shape (which gave them their other name—torpedo bras). Bullet bras aren't really worn on a day-to-day basis anymore, but they are essential for pinup or retro fashions. Many people find them to be quite supportive as well, especially if they don't like underwires. Bullet bras are one of the few styles that can provide significant lift and shaping (although a very specific shape) without an underwire. Those with shallower or full-on-bottom bust shapes may find they need to use bullet bra pads to entirely fill out the cup.

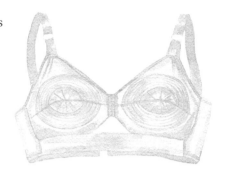

Bustier

Bustiers, also known as basques, are a modern-day version of the corset. Bustiers lift the bust, shape the waist, and smooth the tummy, usually with the assistance of metal or plastic boning. Extremely supportive, especially for all-day wear, bustiers are popular among brides as the undergarment of choice beneath wedding dresses. Because bustiers distribute the weight of the bust along a greater surface area (think of it as an extra-long band . . . and most of the support for your bra comes from the band), they're a wonderful option for people with especially heavy busts. (See chapter 3 for more waist-cinching and body-shaping options.)

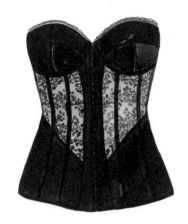

Contour Cup/T-Shirt

The most popular bra style today, the contour cup, or T-shirt bra, consists of seamless, rounded, machine-molded cups made from foam (hence its other name—molded cup bra). T-shirt bras are usually, but not always, lined or slightly padded; they're meant to shape and contour the bust, not add bulk. Contour cups both hide the nipples and disguise uneven breasts, giving a completely smooth silhouette under clothing. Contour cups are a versatile,

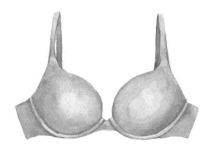

all-around option for a wide range of sizes and situations. However, people with soft breasts may find they're not able to fill the entire cup, and those with larger or heavier breasts will get more support from a cut-and-sew bra.

Cut-and-Sew

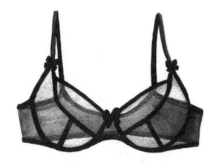

Also known as seamed bras, cut-and-sew bras are made from multiple pieces of fabric that are cut and stitched in such a way that they shape and support the breasts. The most popular version of the cut-and-sew is called a three-part cup, so named because the cup is made of three pieces of fabric (usually two at the bottom and one at the top). Seamed bras come in a wider range of colors and fabrics than molded cup bras. This is the most supportive bra style, and it offers the greatest range of sizes, as well as the most options for shaping the bust. These bras are good at centering and uplifting the breast tissue, especially for people whose breasts splay or point outward. Seamed bras also provide structure and stability for softer or more pendulous breasts. Finally, seams strengthen and reinforce the cup shape, which makes this style perfect for heavy or large breasts. The biggest potential drawback is that the seams may show through clothing. However, some brands now lay fabric atop the seams to give the illusion and wearability of a seamless bra, while providing the structure of a cut-and-sew underneath.

Demi

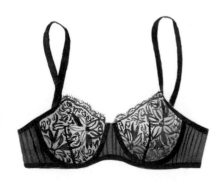

Translating to "half" in French, demi cup bras cover about half the breast, giving less coverage than a full cup bra but more coverage than a balconette or quarter cup bra. Demi bras are one of the most popular bra styles, as well as my personal favorite style, as they offer a nice balance of coverage and support. Because of their lower-cut neckline, demi cups work well with an incredibly wide variety of tops and dresses. Demi bras are a versitile option for a range of bust shapes, including shallow and full-on-bottom shapes (and are especially useful if you're not quite sure of your shape!).

Frame

Frame bras consist of elastic or ribbon sewn into a triangle cup bra shape . . . but surprise! There's no actual fabric to cover the cups. Frame bras give no support and even less coverage, but they do attractively frame the breasts. A popular option for the boudoir or for special occasions, frame bras leave absolutely nothing to the imagination.

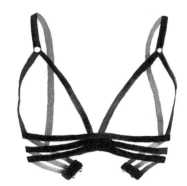

Front Closure

A front closure bra does exactly what the name suggests—it swaps the traditional back hook-and-eye closure for a zipper, clasp, or hook-and-eye closure on the front of the bra. In terms of fashion, front closure bras are popular because they make the back of the bra entirely smooth. This style works well for people with widely spaced breasts, but the closure may rest uncomfortably atop the breast tissue for those with closely spaced breasts. Front closure bras are also useful to people with dexterity or mobility concerns, as the front closures may be easier to handle than rear closures. However, front closure bras often don't fit quite as well and are not quite as supportive as bras with a traditional back closure, since the center panel or gore may not anchor as closely to the body (see page 34 to learn why it's important for the center panel to rest flat atop your breastbone). In addition, front closure bras offer less fit adjustability. They usually have only a single column of closures at the front, as opposed to the multiple columns of back closure bras, which allows for the band to be tightened or loosened.

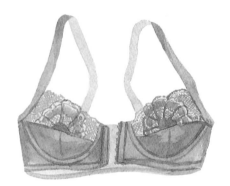

Full Coverage

A full coverage or full cup bra covers most of the breast. This style tends to be extremely supportive (especially for larger busts) and helps create a smooth line under shirts (especially when made from molded cups or seamless fabrics), because

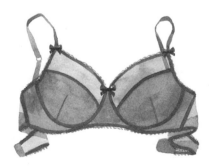

there's no seam cutting across the top of the breast tissue, as in demi or balconette cups. Full coverage bras are perfect for full-all-around breasts, but full-on-bottom or shallow breasts may have difficulty filling out the cups.

Longline

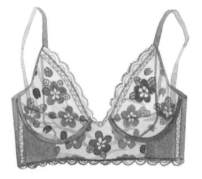

A longline bra has an extended band. The word *longline* refers only to the band, so these bras can have any type of cup shape and style—strapless, plunge, balconette, bralette, contour, cut-and-sew, and so on. It may help to think of a longline as a shorter bustier; some people even call these midi bras. Instead of ending around the fullest part of the rib cage, a longline bra band extends to the bottom of the ribs or even as far as the waist. Longline bras are often used in combination with a fabric called *power mesh* (a strong, stretchy type of mesh popular in lingerie). They're especially good at smoothing out lines under clothing. People with fuller busts may find that longline bras are more supportive, as they distribute the weight of the breasts over a larger area. However, people with flared rib cages or a broad, muscular back may find longline bras uncomfortable.

Mastectomy

Mastectomy bras are designed specifically for people who have undergone a mastectomy, or surgical removal of the breasts. People who have undergone a lumpectomy or partial breast removal may also prefer mastectomy bras. The key distinguishing feature of a mastectomy bra is a pocket or pockets for a breast prosthesis. Mastectomy bras feature other important characteristics as well, such as soft inner linings and an absence of underwires. (For more information on post-mastectomy bra shopping, see page 124.)

Maternity & Nursing

Maternity and nursing bras are made for those who are pregnant and/or nursing. The two terms are often used interchangeably, but maternity bras are specifically worn during pregnancy and may have size-flexible cups, which stretch as your breasts grow to accommodate a period of intense breast growth and change, while nursing bras are worn after the baby is born and have clasps to free the nipple to give better access for feeding. Most, but not all, nursing and maternity bras are wireless. Because these bra styles are meant to be extra comfortable and flexible, they're also good for people who aren't pregnant but whose breasts fluctuate in size often, as well as for people with skin sensitivity concerns or conditions such as fibromyalgia.

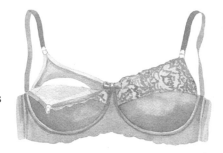

Minimizing

Minimizer bras create the illusion of a smaller bust by reducing breast projection. Minimizer bras don't actually shrink your breasts; the effect is usually achieved by flattening the breasts and pressing them toward the sides of the body. While minimizer bras are a popular style for larger breasts, the same effect can be achieved (minus the squishing) by wearing a more supportive bra in the appropriate size.

Multiway or Convertible

Multiway or convertible bras have removable and adjustable straps that can be worn in a halter, racerback, strapless, or one-shoulder configuration. Some convertible bras also have adjustable bands, allowing the bra to be modified for low-back or backless styles. A convertible bra is a great investment, especially if you have a number of "tricky" wardrobe pieces; they help ensure you'll be well-supported no matter what you wear!

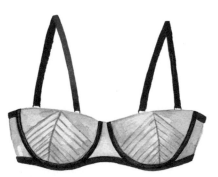

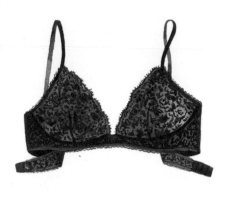

Plunge

My second-favorite bra style, plunge bras are recognized by their deep, low-cut, V neckline. The center panel or gore of a plunge bra tends to be very narrow, and many plunge bras have push-up pads (usually placed along the bottom and outer edges of the cups) to help push the breasts together and create cleavage. Backless/strapless or "invisible" bra styles (such as certain types of adhesive bras) also tend to utilize the plunge silhouette. Plunge bras often aren't a good fit for pendulous or soft breasts, as the smaller cup area means the breasts can fall out of the center of the bra. However, plunge bras are excellent under low necklines. The deepest plunge styles are called *u-plunges*.

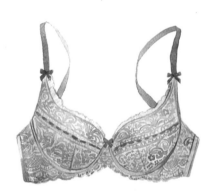

Push-up

One of the most famous bra styles (after a certain lingerie brand popularized them with a memorably "angelic" ad campaign), push-up bras are usually a demi or plunge shape but with significant foam (and sometimes air, gel, or even water) padding on the interior of the cup to add volume and give a fuller bust profile. *Cookies* and other bra inserts are a type of removable push-up padding. While many people assume only those with smaller bra sizes would want to wear push-ups, they're suitable and popular for a wide range of bra sizes. Push-up bras are also a good option to give shallower breast shapes the appearance of a fuller bust.

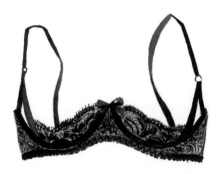

Quarter Cup or Shelf

Between the balconette bra and the frame bra is the quarter cup bra. Consisting of just enough cup fabric to support and lift the breasts from beneath and no more, quarter cup bras are a popular boudoir option. Some companies combine the frame bra's silhouette with the quarter cup bra shape for maximum display. Quarter cup bras may be made from lace, mesh, or even foam. Other names for this bra include open cup, cupless, and chopper.

Sports

Sports bras are made for athletic activity. They're meant to protect the breasts and the surrounding ligaments from excessive bouncing and movement. Sports bras help to reduce pain and strain during physical activity and can eliminate bruising, chafing, and skin irritation. They are available for a variety of workout intensity levels, ranging from those suitable for low-impact activities (such as yoga) to high-impact activities (such as running). Sports bras tend to fall into two main styles: compression and encapsulated. The first works by pressing the breasts to the chest and is good for smaller busts, while the latter has two separate, often underwired, cups and gives better support for larger busts. Sports bras can also be used as binders or chest minimizers. However, it's important to buy a sports bra in the appropriate size: too large and the sports bra won't be able to effectively minimize bounce; too small and the extra constriction may injure your soft tissues.

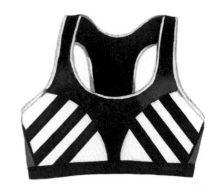

Strapless

As the name suggests, a strapless bra is a bra without straps. It can be contour cup, cut-and-sew, or even bandeau style—the only requirement being a lack of straps. Many strapless bras utilize silicone or adhesive to help the bra stay in place. Bustier or longline strapless styles will be the most supportive for heavier busts; the wide band provides a better anchor, which allows for more support. Strapless bra styles work beautifully for strapless tops and dresses, of course, but are also ideal for asymmetrical, halter neck, or spaghetti strap tops.

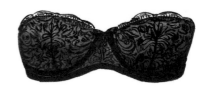

Surgery

These bras are worn after procedures like breast augmentation, lumpectomy, and mastectomy. Post-surgery bras are better for this purpose than sports bras or wirefree bralettes, as they're specially developed to give support and allow freedom of movement, while reducing pressure on sensitive tissues. Post-surgery bras can also help with edema (swelling), and certain styles have special pouches or pockets to assist with medical fluids or drainage. For this kind of bra, it's especially important to check in with your doctor, who will have the best information on the specific style or type you'll need.

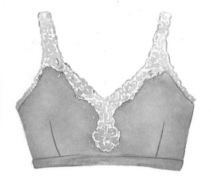

Wireless

Wireless bras, also known as wirefree or soft cup bras, do not have underwires. Because the underwire is what gives structure and shape to a traditional bra, bras without underwires (such as bralettes or sports bras) are rarely able to give the same amount of lift. Wirefree bras tend to be popular as sleep or lounge bras and also as mastectomy or maternity bras, as underwires can be irritating to sensitive tissues.

How to Find Your Perfect Bra Fit

Bra fit, like bra sizing, can be very complicated and full of nuance and exceptions and special cases. Why? Because all bodies are different, and it's impossible to say what will work for every single person, every single time. Rather than giving you a list of rules, I want to give you a set of fundamentals to help you understand how a well-fitting bra should feel. Once you know these, it's not only easier to discover your perfect, personalized fit but you'll also be able to find the best bras for your body, no matter the brand, size, or style.

- **Center gore:** In underwired styles, the center gore should lie flat against your breastbone with no gaps or spaces. This is called *tacking*. The gore also shouldn't feel like a seesaw, that is, digging in one side more than the other. When a gore tacks, it anchors the bra against your sternum, helping to keep it firm, stable, and in place all day. People with close-set breasts (for example, one finger width apart), may have trouble finding a bra with a gore that tacks; look for plunge and other deep styles to address that issue. Wireless bras will never have a tacking gore; however, the band should still lie flat against the body.

- **Cups:** The underwires (if present) should completely surround the breasts at the crease where your breasts meet your chest. There shouldn't be any breast tissue escaping outside, over, or under the cup. You can test this for underwired bras by pressing along the outside edge of the wire while wearing the bra; your fingers should be pressing over your rib cage, not the breast itself. For wirefree styles, you want to ensure that your breasts are fully contained within the seams or cup area, not spilling into or under the band or bulging out of the cups. Whether it's an underwire or wireless style, you should feel fully contained within the cups. If not, you may not have your best fit.

- **Band:** The band, which provides the majority of the support for your bra, needs to be completely horizontal. A band should neither ride up nor dip down, and you shouldn't be able to stretch it more than a few inches from the body. A well-fitting band is firm, like a hug, but not so tight it hurts, bruises, or cuts into the skin. It may sound counterintuitive, but a tighter band is more supportive than a looser band; the band needs to grip the body in order to work. Some people may find that their bra leaves marks, such as small indentations in the shape of the band, after wear. While this is normal (because our skin is flexible), bruises, welts, red marks that don't go away, rashes, broken skin, and pain are not normal and mean that there is either an issue with your bra (such as an allergic reaction) or that you're wearing a bra that's not a good size or shape for you.

In addition to these three ways of checking for good fit, look at the straps (do they dig into or fall off the shoulders?), the top of the cups (does your breast tissue fall over the top edge or is there a gap?), and the cup itself (does it dimple, pucker, or wrinkle?).

If you find your bra doesn't fit as well as it could or should, following are a few quick fixes to try.

STAYING CENTERED: HOW TO "SWOOP AND SCOOP"

To ensure the best fit and support, use the "swoop and scoop" method to center your breasts within your bra cups.

- With your bra on, lean forward as far as is comfortable.

- One side at a time, grab the outside edge of the bra with the hand on the same side (so left side, left hand; right side, right hand).

- Using the opposite hand, cup the far side of the breast (near the armpit) and scoop it toward the center, pulling the entirety of the breast into the cup. You may need to lift the breast slightly to make sure it's fully seated within the curve of the underwire.

- After centering both breasts, straighten up and double check that your breasts are completely contained and lifted within the cups. You may need to repeat the process, which is normal. Practice makes perfect!

Sometimes a bra will fit less well after swooping and scooping. Don't panic! See page 17 to learn more about finding your best fit.

LINED, UNLINED, AND PADDED CUPS

When it comes to padding, bras can be divided into three major categories—lined, unlined, and padded.

Lined: Lined bras contain a very thin layer of foam within the cups. This foam shapes or contours the breasts, which is why lined bras are also known as contour cup bras. In addition to helping give both breasts an identical, uniform shape, lined cups also shield or hide the nipples and help give a smooth look under clothing. Lined bras are almost always molded cups instead of cut-and-sew, although some styles are a molded/cut-and-sew hybrid where the foam itself is stitched into the shape of a multipart cup. More frequently, however, there will be a faux cut-and-sew effect on the top of the cup for aesthetics, while the interior of the cup is a single, molded piece of foam. The key difference between a contour cup and a padded cup is that a contour cup gives shape and definition without adding bulk or volume.

Unlined: Usually made from one or two layers of lace, mesh, embroidery, or knit fabric, an unlined cup contains no padding or foam. Unlined cups tend to be very light and airy, which make them ideal for warmer months. The cup itself is also very soft and flexible; unlike the cup for a T-shirt bra, it won't take a shape until it's actually placed on the body. Many cut-and-sew styles, as well as many bralettes, tend to be unlined. Unlined bras can be very comfortable, but their biggest downside is they offer no extra nipple coverage They're also not a good fit for people who want the added shaping and lift of a contour cup or push-up bra.

Padded: Padded bras add noticeable size and definition to the breasts, with the most dramatic padded styles promising an increase of two cup sizes or more. Push-up bras are a specific type of padded bra; the padding is concentrated along the sides and/or bottom of the cup to lift up the breasts and push them together. Padded bras are great for uneven breasts or for times a person just wants "more up there." However, they can be very warm, especially if the pads aren't removable, and they also require extra care when washing and drying so the padding doesn't lose its shape or become deformed. (See pages 109–114 for more information on washing bras and the bonus tip on page 38 for how to reshape a dented or warped molded cup.)

- **If your bra band rides up in the back,** that usually means it's too loose. Try going down a band size (for example, from a 38 to a 36). Also, make sure your straps aren't overly tight, as that could be pulling your band up in the back. Finally, look into bras with a leotard or u-back or with longline bands to provide more secure placement and better anchoring. If you can't find a small enough band for your cup volume, look into a band shortener, like the Rixie Clip.

- **If your bra band feels too tight** (for example, it's leaving bruises or raw places), go up a band size (such as from a 34 to a 36). If you can't find a band size large enough for your cup volume, try a band extender.

- **If the straps dig into your shoulders,** first make sure they're not too tight (remember: the majority of support should come from the band, not the straps). If that doesn't work, sister size down one band and up one cup size, as your band may be too loose, which means your straps are working too hard. If that's not an option, look into padded or cushioned straps. Wider straps also tend to be more comfortable than narrower straps, as the weight they support is spread over a larger area.

- **If your straps fall off your shoulders,** they may be too widely spaced for you. Consider using a racerback bra-strap converter, especially if you have smaller, narrower shoulders. A leotard or u-back, as mentioned earlier, is also a good idea for small shoulders. You might try sizing down a band (a band that's too big could make the straps too widely spaced for your body).

- **If the center gore won't tack,** that is, lie flat against your sternum, the cups may be too small or not deep enough for you. Try a larger cup size (and remember that you can also try your sister size—a larger cup size with a smaller band size!). If you have narrowly spaced breasts, look for bras with a low center panel, like a plunge style. Remember, however, that wireless styles are not designed to lie flat. Tacking is for underwires.

- **If your breasts are bulging out of the cups,** often there's a mismatch between the bra shape and your breast shape. Try a different bra shape (for example, a full-coverage style instead

of a demi). If you find the spillage happens on the sides, look into bras with a side sling or side boning to pull your breast tissue front and center, or consider going up a cup size.

- **If your breasts can't seem to fill out the cups**, there may also be a mismatch between your breast shape and the cup shape. Try a different bra shape (for example, a plunge or balconette instead of a full-coverage style, so there's less bra) or consider sister sizing down a cup size.

The most important thing to remember is that nothing replaces trial and error. No amount of reading, of this book or any other, can take the place of trying on bras and seeing how they work for you. I know that it can be frustrating, tedious, and even expensive, but while there are ways to make the learning process easier (such as by reading reviews from lingerie bloggers or taking advantage of free-shipping offers), nothing and no one can replace knowing how a bra fits on *you*.

In addition, if a bra doesn't work for you, that's not a sign there's anything wrong with your body. There are lots of different kinds of normal, and so bras have to be made with lots of little variations to accommodate as many people as possible. Otherwise, we'd all have to buy custom lingerie! Fit can change slightly between brands, styles, and even colorways, so think of it as an opportunity to have fun and experiment! Oh, and don't forget to stock up once you find your "holy grail" bra! There's nothing worse than discovering a new fave only to have it discontinued.

Finally, please keep in mind that bra size is not static. Menstrual cycles, birth control, weight loss or gain, hormone treatments, menopause, pregnancy, nursing, and age can and will affect your breast size and how your bras fit. It is common—and can be very helpful—to have more than one size in your lingerie drawer, not just because of those size inconsistences between brands I mentioned before but also because you may prefer different sizes at different times of the month. That's normal and okay. As always, what counts most is buying what's comfortable for you. Just don't get discouraged before finding your perfect bra!

BONUS TIP

To reshape a dented bra cup, soak it in hot water, reshaping the cup with your fingers. For stubborn dents, wearing your damp bra until it dries or filling the cups with heavy silicone inserts will help to flatten out the depressions.

Bra Prices & What They Tell You

Bra prices can range from $5 to $500. While it makes intuitive sense that a more expensive bra is likely to be of higher quality and have better construction than a cheaper bra, what exactly do you get for your money?

The first thing to know is that fabrics and materials make up a relatively small portion of bra prices. Labor (designers, pattern graders, fabric cutters, sewists, etc.) is by far the biggest expense, and cheap bras are usually cheaper because they've been made in places where the cost to employ people is low.

Labor costs are also why bras for larger busts often cost more than bras for smaller busts. The amount of work involved in making them—from research and development to construction costs—is significantly higher, especially since the bra is doing more work by holding up more weight. However, there are noticeable differences in quality between a cheap bra and a more expensive bra. Let's break it down.

- **Less expensive bras** (under $40) tend to be plain, simple styles made from lower-quality materials. For example, a bra in this price range will likely have plastic clips and adjusters instead of metal ones. In addition, the fabric may feel stiff and rough or the elastic may be overly stretchy. For ultra-cheap bras, such as those costing $10 or less, you might even notice signs of shoddy construction, like loose threads and irregular stitching. The bra will still work, more or less, but it probably won't last very long and will need replacing much sooner than a higher-quality bra.

- **Around the $45 price mark** and ranging up until the $90 to $100 mark, there's an abrupt change in both quality and aesthetics. I call this the bra-shopping sweet spot. The price is high enough to notice a real difference in the value you get for your money but still low enough to be accessible to the average person (especially during sale season; flip to page 5 to see when the best lingerie sales happen). This price point is where you'll start to see more expensive, better-quality fabrics (such as delicate laces) as well as time-intensive construction techniques, like cut-and-sew. These bras might also include beautiful little details like lacy straps, delicate bows, and elegant embroidery, or more practical materials like spacer fabric (a highly breathable, lightweight textile that supports the breasts while keeping them cool).

- **If you're able to spend $100 or more on a bra,** you'll see some truly amazing works of art. The three-figure mark is when brands go all out to create incredibly special pieces of lingerie using the most beautiful, luxurious, and unique fabrics. At this price point, materials like silk satin, silk tulle, Chantilly lace, guipure (a type of lace), and *broderie anglaise* (eyelet lace) are common, as are custom prints and embroideries and even bras that use multiple laces on a single cup. Bras at this price point may also have custom-designed hardware, like strap adjusters with the company's logo (sometimes dipped in 24-karat gold!), and thoughtful design details like cushioned underwires or a velvet-lined band.

When to Get Rid of a Bra

A dead bra doesn't do you or your breasts any favors. While some experts recommend replacing your bra every six months, I'm more of the mindset that you should just pay attention to when your bra isn't doing its job anymore. If you know what signs to look for, you'll be ready to give your old bras the boot when it's time.

- **The bra elastic is worn out**. Because most of the support comes from the band, if your band loses its elasticity, your bra can't do its job. Similarly, if your bra straps are stretched out and won't stay in place no matter what, it's time to toss it.

- **The bra is dingy, faded, and discolored**. Your bra is probably the first thing you put on in the morning and the last thing you take off at night. It's against your skin all day. It affects the way your clothes look and fit but, most important, it affects how you feel. You deserve to wear something nice against your body. Throw out that old, tired-looking bra.

- **The bra is misshapen, torn, or has missing or crooked underwires.** If you have to basically rebuild your bra after every wear (or if it's trying to stab you in the heart), throw it out. A good bra feels effortless; you should forget it as soon as you put it on. You can't do that if it's falling to pieces.

- **The bra just doesn't feel right or makes you feel bad.** If your bra is uncomfortable, itchy, chafing, or just plain makes you feel depressed every time you look at it, get rid of it. Don't tell yourself you'll love it one day or that you'll eventually get around to wearing it more. That bra won't get any better, and it won't make you feel any better. Don't punish yourself with a bad bra.

Just in case you need one final push, you have my permission to treat yourself to a new bra you love and one that you're excited about wearing! You deserve it!

BONUS TIP

If your bra wires feel too tight or painful, try putting a bit of moleskin between the wire and your skin. You can also try bending the wire into a better shape for your body with pliers. Moleskin is also useful if your underwire pops out. Just slide the wire back into the channel and put a small piece of moleskin over the tear. A dab of superglue can help this fix last longer. Find adhesive moleskin in the foot-care aisle of a drugstore.

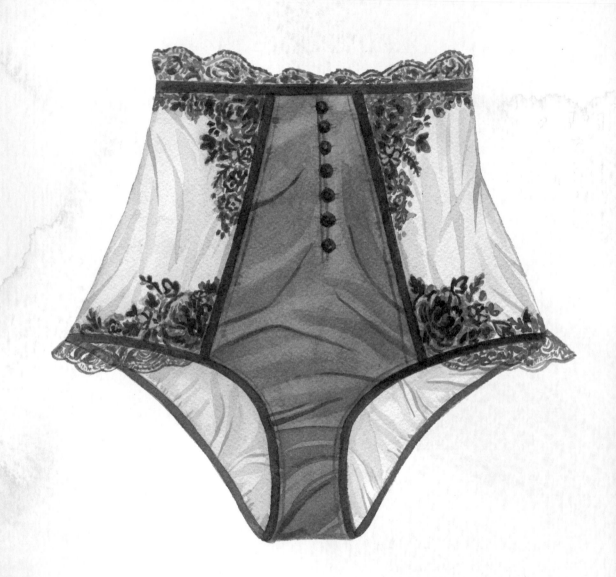

CHAPTER 2

UNDERWEAR

We all know there's good underwear and there's bad underwear. The good stuff makes your life easier, but the bad stuff . . . well, is there anything worse than being stuck in a pair of undies that makes you miserable?

Good underwear is about more than invisible panty lines or a shapely derriere; it's about making you feel great and preparing you to tackle the day, no matter what it has in store. While underwear is a basic item of lingerie, knowing how to shop for it can be empowering. I talk to so many people who feel like there's simply no good underwear out there for them, when usually the truth is they just don't yet have the vocabulary to describe the kind of underwear they're looking for—it's hard to find something you can't name. Good underwear lets you be the best version of yourself, and we can all use some of that.

A Brief History of Underwear

While undergarments like loincloths have existed for most of human history, underwear as we think of it today was first worn by European women in the eighteenth century. Many historians believe that before then, women simply didn't wear anything beneath their chemises. However, thoughts on women's fashion are always changing, and a few historians now believe women wore *braes* (what we might think of as boxer shorts today) under their gowns. I have to admit that considering certain factors like menstruation and post-pregnancy bleeding, wearing some type of underwear at least some of the time seems logical.

In the days of stays, farthingales, petticoats, and bum rolls (all types of sixteenth-century lingerie), an extra layer in the form of drawers must have seemed preposterous. Why wear yet another undergarment designed specifically to cover one's private areas if they're already hidden by layers and layers of heavy skirts?

Bifurcated or divided garments (like pants or boxer shorts) were seen as masculine. The idea of a woman wearing trousers or breeches, even invisibly beneath a dress, was thought to be a violation of the natural order of things. While there are some historical reports of Italian women wearing drawers (described as silk or linen breeches under their gowns) in the seventeenth century, the trend for women's underwear doesn't appear to have caught on and become widespread at this time.

Sometime between the eighteenth and nineteenth centuries, as skirts shortened slightly and mass production became more feasible, women began to wear pantalettes or pantaloons beneath their dresses. As an aside, this is where the rather unpopular American word *panties* comes from (and likely also its U.K. equivalent, *pants*).

The development of the cage crinoline in the mid-nineteenth century—a lightweight understructure that replaced heavier petticoats (and was vulnerable to sudden gusts of wind)—sealed the introduction of underwear into the intimate wardrobes of women. No matter how inappropriate people may have thought underwear was a century or two before, it was certainly more appropriate than the possibility of revealing one's nether regions on a windy day.

These first pairs of underwear consisted of two separate legs joined at the waist with buttons or laces. Because drawers (so named because they were drawn up the body) were literally a pair of legs, we still refer to underwear today as a "pair" of panties.

One interesting (and possibly scandalous) fact about early underwear: It was all completely open in the middle—what we might call *ouvert*, or "open gusset," today. At the time, this was seen as hygienic, particularly for using the loo, but it was also seen as more modest and appropriate, a sharp departure from how people nowadays view crotchless knickers!

Trends in lingerie are often closely linked to trends in outerwear, and after the Victorian and Edwardian Eras, lingerie changed again. First, as skirts and dresses slimmed down in the 1870s (the sleek princess-style gown, worn by Princess Alexandra, was popular), drawers became sleeker and less voluminous as well. Combinations that further cut down on bulk, such as chemises with drawers, also debuted during this era.

After World War I, the streamlining of women's underwear continued. This was the flapper generation, and shorter hems required closed-crotch knickers. Tap pants and camiknickers (the first a shorter version of pantalettes and the second an all-in-one garment combining a camisole with tap shorts) appeared first. These gradually shortened into the familiar high-waisted briefs of the 1940s and 1950s. Lavishly ruffled knickers and underwear with kitschy embroidery (such as the days of the week) were also popular during this time.

During the 1960s and 1970s, as hemlines and waistlines fell, lower-cut and less-full-coverage hipster or bikini styles appeared. Both these types of underwear were popular because of their minimal coverage, which meant minimal visibility under miniskirts and tight clothing.

According to some fashion historians, the thong was also invented in the 1970s, by Rudi Gernreich. However, others credit Frederick Mellinger, the founder of Frederick's of Hollywood, with inventing the thong in the 1980s. If nothing else, Frederick's mail-order catalogs certainly helped make it more popular! I prefer to credit vintage burlesque dancers and showgirls, who have been wearing G-strings and thongs since at least the 1920s and 1930s (in order to get around nudity laws), for its invention.

The 1980s was an era of strong silhouettes and "power dressing," and brought the lingerie world such classics as string bikinis and super-high-cut underwear. In the 1990s, thongs reigned supreme thanks to Hanky Panky, a brand that popularized stretch lace underwear. Later, in the 2000s, cheeky, boyshort, and Brazilian-cut panties, preferably with super-low, below-the-hip-bone rises, were all the rage.

And today? Well, briefs and other full-coverage styles are making a comeback, but we're lucky to live in an era where people can wear whatever they want and where advances in technology—such as laser-cut seams, moisture-wicking fabrics, and tagless underwear—mean the dreaded visible panty line is a ghost of knickers past.

WHAT IS "RISE"?

In the simplest terms, an underwear's *rise* refers to how high up the body the waistband comes. The very highest rises are above the navel, at the natural waist, or even higher (as in certain types of shaping briefs that can reach up to the rib cage). The very lowest rises dip as far down as the pubic bone. Most underwear is somewhere between these two extremes with what's called either a moderate or low rise that usually ends somewhere between the navel and hip bones.

Why Underwear?

Though many people think of underwear as something necessary for health reasons, the truth is that underwear, like most lingerie, is more about protecting our clothing and providing coverage and comfort than about hygiene. The original purpose of underwear, apart from shaping the body, was to protect expensive, delicate fabrics. In a time when even the simplest clothing represented many, many hours of hand labor and when almost nothing could be washed, shielding clothing from the natural oils, perspirations, and fluids of the body was very important.

Modern-day underwear accomplishes the same task. Knickers protect your outerwear from the natural scents and secretions of the human body. That said, like a lot of lingerie-related matters, the decision to wear underwear is entirely personal, and you should do what feels best for you and works best for your body.

Types of Underwear

From ethically produced briefs to bikinis made from recycled plastics to ultra-fabulous, limited-edition silk tap pants to straightforward cotton hipsters sold by the six-pack, we are inundated with underwear choices. Here are the most popular underwear styles for your consideration.

Bikini

Bikinis are characterized by a low rise, often several inches below the belly button, with narrower sides (like a bikini bathing suit). Bikinis can be full coverage in the back (that is, cover the entire derriere) or have a more modern and revealing cheeky cut. Bikinis with the very narrowest sides, usually made of a simple piece of elastic connecting the front and back and nothing more, are called string bikinis.

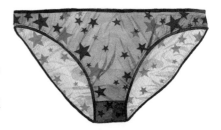

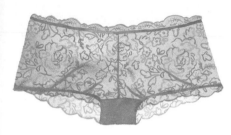

Boyshorts/Women's Boxers

Cut in the style of a traditional masculine boxer brief, but tailored to a more feminine silhouette, boyshorts are distinguished from tap pants by their more tightly fitting legs. Some boyshorts are literal shorts with both full rear coverage and extended upper thigh coverage. Other boyshorts are cut in a cheeky style, with shorter legs partially revealing the derriere. Generally speaking, underwear labeled *boyshorts* will give slightly less coverage than underwear with the name *boxers*.

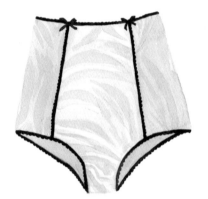

Briefs

Often consisting of a high-waisted front and full-coverage back with either low or high leg openings, briefs have a vintage pinup vibe and were at their most popular during the 1950s and 1980s. Traditional briefs are usually made from fibers like nylon or cotton, while more modern briefs rely on seamless microfibers. Because of their full-coverage rear, briefs are excellent for avoiding visible panty lines, especially for people who'd rather not wear thongs.

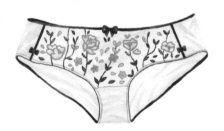

Hipster

A hipster is a hybrid style somewhere between a bikini, boyshort, and brief. Hipsters have a lower rise than a brief (usually at right around the hip bones, hence the name) but a higher rise than a traditional bikini. From the front, a hipster's wider sides resemble a boyshort. However, the back coverage is more akin to a bikini. Hipsters are a great way to get a little more coverage without the added bulk or height of a boyshort or brief.

Tanga/Brazilian

Another hybrid style, a tanga, or Brazilian panty, is a cross between a bikini and a thong. Tangas give bikini-style coverage in the front and narrow, cheeky coverage in the back—covering more than a thong but considerably less than a brief.

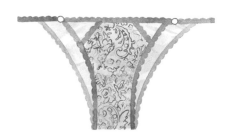

Tap Pants/Tap Shorts

A loose-cut short covering the upper portion of the thigh as well as the hips and derriere, this vintage style was first made popular in the 1920s. In the modern era, the tap short is a wonderful alternative for people who find "regular" underwear too tight or clingy. Tap shorts are also a good option for people who prefer wearing dresses and skirts but want more coverage than modern underwear typically provides. Tap shorts differ from boxer briefs in that they have a looser, more fluttery cut. Tap pants may also be called culottes or French knickers.

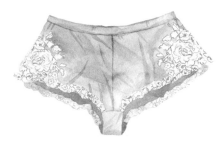

Thong

The thong panty is designed to leave the bottom more or less uncovered. Thongs usually have a bikini-style front (like both the bikini and tanga styles mentioned previously), however the back is a narrow strip of fabric meant to be seated between the cheeks (as opposed to covering them). The very skimpiest thongs are called G-strings, where the back of the panty is simply a string around the waist and another string between the bottom cheeks.

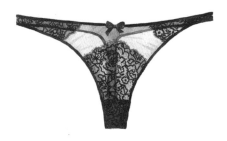

Other Types of Underwear

These include the garter panty (simply a panty with garters for attaching stockings), the C-string (a type of flexible thong without sides that tucks against the body), and pettipants (which are old-school pantalettes that can be worn in lieu of a slip and underwear).

Underwear Fibers

Fabric is just as important as fit and style when you're talking underwear. Some fabrics and fibers are more comfortable than others, especially if you have a skin sensitivity or allergy. Some fibers are also better at functions like moisture wicking or breathability, which is very important when you're considering which underwear to choose.

Following is a list of the most popular fiber choices for underwear and a few of their respective strengths and weaknesses. These fibers are also used in many other types of lingerie, so keep this section handy as a reference when you're ready to shop. Any of the underwear styles mentioned previously can be made with any of the following fibers.

Bamboo

Bamboo is an amazingly soft, absorbent, sweat-wicking fiber that, like silk, is warm in the winter and cool in the summer. Some also believe bamboo has antibacterial properties, although the research is inconclusive. Despite its many positive characteristics, bamboo is not quite as durable as cotton and tends to be more expensive than almost any other underwear fiber (with the exception of silk).

Cotton

Cotton feels fresh and cool against the skin and is easily washable and highly breathable. However, a major downside of cotton is that it's incredibly absorbent and can hold a lot of moisture, which can make the material feel wet and soggy against the skin (not to mention creating a good environment for moisture irritation or infection). Cotton fibers can also lose their shape after a while, especially if they've been treated harshly (as in machine washed and tumble dried!).

Nylon

Soft, water-repellent, easy to wash, easy to store, and difficult to wrinkle, artificial-fiber nylon holds it shape well and lasts for a long time. However, nylon is neither absorbent nor breathable, which can lead to moisture "puddling" in warmer weather (in addition to the possibility of fungal or bacterial infections). Nylon is a strong and versatile fiber, often making its way into fabrics such as satin, tulle, mesh, and lace.

Polyester

Another water-repellent artificial fiber, polyester can take on the sheen of satin or the softness of microfiber. Many technical blends (fabrics with enhanced properties such as moisture wicking or thermal insulation) are made from polyester, which means polyester is perfect for activewear, like sports and leggings. Polyester is both strong and durable. However, once a scent or stain gets embedded in the fibers, it can be difficult, if not impossible, to wash out.

Rayon

Also known as modal or viscose, rayon is soft and cool to the touch, and the very best grades of rayon can feel almost like silk (in fact, rayon was marketed as "artificial silk" in the early twentieth century). Like bamboo, rayon is a plant-based textile, and many people find rayon to be just as, if not more, breathable than cotton. However, rayon is not as strong as nylon, cotton, or even silk and tends to lose its shape and degrade over time.

Silk

Favored by royals and commoners alike, silk is a luxurious fiber made exclusively by silkworms. Silk is soft, strong, breathable, cool in the summer, and warm in the winter. It also wicks away moisture easily and is naturally hypoallergenic. Finally, silk has a beautiful natural luster no other fiber can imitate. However, silk is incredibly expensive and requires special care and handling. Hand washing (see pages 110–111) or even dry cleaning (see pages 114–115) is mandatory, lest you permanently ruin the delicate fibers. Because authentic silk is always an animal product, it may not be suitable for vegans.

Spandex

Also known as LYCRA and elastane, spandex is far stronger than its predecessor, rubber. Almost anything with stretch contains at least a little bit of spandex. Shapewear tends to be made with the most spandex (the elastic fibers both help to shape the body and keep the garment from being stretched out of shape, otherwise known as *recovery*), but almost all modern-day underwear contains some. A strong, lightweight fiber, spandex helps undergarments stretch to fit the body without bagginess. However, spandex is susceptible to heat and degrades quickly with machine drying or ironing. It's also not absorbent and can lead to skin irritation issues, similar to nylon and polyester.

Other Less-Common Underwear Fibers

These include wool, linen, acrylic, soy, hemp, and even latex and leather (which are technically materials, not fibers).

How to Find Your Perfect Underwear Fit

I've said it before, but I think it's really important to say again: the kind of underwear you prefer and how you want it to fit is entirely personal; only you know what works best for your body. So think of this section as offering a few suggestions or tips to keep in mind, *not* a list of hard-and-fast rules.

No matter what, your underwear should be comfortable enough to wear all day (and for whatever task you choose to do, whether that's running a marathon or running errands). Your underwear should not hurt or harm your body, which I know seems obvious but I've talked to so many people who expect their underwear to be painful, and it shouldn't be. If your underwear twists, digs, binds, chafes, causes bruises, infections, or pain, then it's not the right underwear for you. You deserve comfy undies!

Remember: It can take a bit of trial and error to find your perfect brand or style, and it's normal for your tastes to change over time. Keep an open mind, be willing to experiment, and don't forget to stock up once you find something you love!

Sizing yourself for underwear requires two measurements: your waist and your hip. As with bras, every brand has its own size chart, so don't forget to check that when trying a new label. A cloth tape measure (*not* the kind you'd use in construction projects), which you can buy from a drugstore, is good to have on hand if you don't know your measurements (or if you suspect they've changed).

When taking your hip measurement, wrap the tape measure around your low hip at its fullest point. For most people, this will be the widest part of their bottom. You want to make sure the tape measure is pulled snugly around the body and that it's horizontal all the way around. However, you don't want to pull so tight that the tape measure digs into your skin; you should be able to fit a fingertip between the tape measure and your body. That way, you know you'll have enough room, or *ease*, to stretch, bend, move, walk, sit, and do all the other things you might want to do in your underwear.

When taking your waist measurement, measure your body at the natural crease that appears when you bend to the side (this is usually just above your navel). As with your hip measurement, make sure the tape measure is horizontal and snug (it shouldn't have any slack), but don't pull so tightly that you indent the skin. And remember: no matter what the numbers on the tape measure say, they're just numbers. They're only tools to help you find your perfect fit—not a judgment on you or your body. Once you have both these measurements, consult the size chart of the brand you want to try.

Other things to remember include the type of seam or edges you want (seamless or laser-cut underwear is especially popular right now and is available in almost every style; they're perfect for avoiding visible panty lines), as well as making sure your underwear has a cotton gusset. The gusset is the lining fabric inside the crotch of your underwear. As mentioned earlier, cotton is breathable and

BONUS TIP

Stocking up on basics? Many stores offer panty deals, such as five for $30 or three for $45. If you find a style you like, this is a great way to make sure you have enough knickers for all occasions!

feels cool against the skin. Gussets made from nylon, polyester, or other synthetic fabrics can hold moisture against your private parts, potentially leading to rashes or infection.

Your underwear, once you find the perfect fit, should be smooth, snug, and symmetrical all the way around. Any bunching, binding, or rolling probably means you don't have your best fit. Similarly, lots of excess fabric bunching in the seat or gusset might mean it's time to try another size or style.

When trying on underwear (always over your own knickers, of course!), move around. Bend to the side, bend to the front, sit down, stand up, and walk around. Problems with underwear tend to reveal themselves quickly with a little bit of movement, and if you notice anything that doesn't feel right, don't buy it! Finally, as with bras, when your underwear starts to look stretched out, discolored, or frayed, it's time to buy a new pair.

Your underwear covers and protects the most delicate areas of your body. It should be soft, comfortable, and easygoing so that you can get on your with your day and focus on the things that really matter. After all, life is too short for terrible underwear.

WEDDING LINGERIE

The lingerie you wear on your wedding day will provide the foundation for your ensemble and is a key part of your total wedding look. It can help smooth, shape, support, or even just lightly skim over your body to help you look and feel your best. Popular choices include bustiers, waist cinchers, shaping thongs, shaping slips, longline bras, strapless bras, and adhesive bras. Your bridal shop consultant or tailor is a great resource for finding your ideal underpinnings, sometimes offering creative solutions—like sewing bra cups directly into a dress bodice.

If you're soon-to-be wed, keep these tips in mind when it's time to shop for your ideal unmentionables.

- Wear what you want: Your wedding day is *your* day, and you should feel comfortable, confident, and gorgeous. Don't wear anything you hate or that makes you uncomfortable.

- Function over form: This is a time to choose comfort and support over aesthetics. Save the glamorous boudoir looks for the wedding night or the honeymoon!

- Consider color: While shades of white, cream, ivory, and skin tone–suitable nude are classic choices, colors like robin's egg blue, blush, and champagne are lovely options too.

- Make sure it works: Try everything on with your entire outfit before the wedding day. After you buy your outfit, take pictures of yourself in it to capture all the details (like how low the back is), and immediately begin the lingerie search. Lingerie retailers with flexible return policies are helpful, since you'll likely want to try on several pieces. If your attire requires alterations, remember to bring your undergarments to every fitting.

- Double-check everything: A few weeks before the wedding, make sure all your lingerie still fits and is comfortable. Sizes can change. We can develop skin sensitivities or allergies (especially in response to stress!). Try on everything again, move around in it, and see how it feels thirty or forty-five minutes later to make sure you're still satisfied.

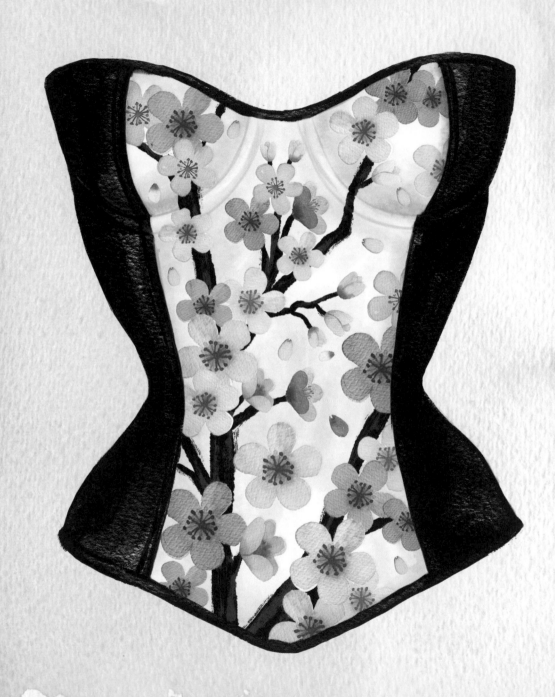

CHAPTER 3

SHAPEWEAR

First things first—nobody *needs* shapewear. While shapewear can help to give a smooth line under clothing, replace traditional underwear, or even, in its most dramatic forms, take an inch or two off your figure, I flatly reject the notion that anybody *has* to wear it. If you want to wear it, that's fine, because lingerie is all about choice. And if you hate it, that's okay too, *because lingerie is all about choice.* You should wear, or not wear, whatever you like.

Shapewear is, at its most basic, a type of lingerie meant to sculpt, smooth, transform, or otherwise mold the figure. Spanx is a type of shapewear, but so is a corset. One is simply more dramatic (and more structured) than the other. The kind of shapewear you choose depends not only upon your personal comfort level but also upon the garment you're wearing. Different pieces—and different degrees of shaping—are best for different kinds of clothing.

While shapewear is often thought of as utilitarian, boring, or even torturous, I believe it can be a fun and fashionable way to experiment with transformation. Shapewear today can lift the bust, nip the waist, and pad the rear, letting you play with proportions and silhouettes that might otherwise require going under the knife. No matter your reason for wearing shapewear, it should help you feel like the best version of yourself. Otherwise, what's the point?

A Brief History of Shapewear

Truthfully, almost all lingerie could be defined as shapewear, and this is especially the case when we look at historical lingerie. In both ancient Greek and Roman culture, a more natural waist was in fashion, and draping fabric loosely around the body to form a garment was the norm. The idea of sculpting the body through fashion didn't appear in Western garments until the Middle Ages.

One major event led to the creation of shapewear: tailoring. While we take seamstresses and tailors for granted today, the rise of tailoring in the thirteenth century led to a shift from draped garments (which we could call *tunics*) to a more body-conscious fit. Clothes for men and women suddenly became tighter, showing the contours and curves of the human form. This newly tightened clothing introduced the concept of figure control.

At first, the trend toward tighter clothing showed itself in tightly sewn or even laced-up bodices. Later, after women's dresses were split into two separate parts (a separate skirt and bodice), these bodices were reinforced with paste, reed, horn, wood, and stiffened rope. All this extra structure eventually migrated underneath the clothing, transforming into stays.

The French took the concept of stays and pushed it even further, exaggerating the ideal of a small waist. Whalebones (actually baleen from inside the mouths of certain whales) became more popular than reeds due to their more effective shaping. Stays were the lingerie de rigueur until the French Revolution.

After the French Revolution, dress waistlines rose to just under the bust (an Empire waist) and stays disappeared. Anything associated with the old regime, including large skirts held out by panniers (a type of hooped petticoat) and artificially small waists, were viewed with suspicion. However, the anti-corset era didn't last long. Less than a generation later, a shortened version of stays, appropriately called *short stays*, arrived. Resembling the modern longline bra, these short stays focused more on lifting the bust than on shaping the waist. Eventually, they lengthened into the first corsets with a shape that resembles a modern-day bustier.

Between the 1830s and 1860s, the tiny waist we now associate with corsets began to emerge, mostly due to technological innovations such as the metal eyelet (which allowed for tighter lacing) and the front split busk (the busk is the metal element at the front of a corset, which helps to keep it both rigid and closed). Corsetry reached its somewhat impractical peak with the S-Curve of the 1900s, a shape that pushed the bust forward and the hips back, resulting in its other name, the pigeon breast (although some experts believe this shape was either created from wholecloth or exaggerated with extra padding).

After World War I, women's fashion transformed. Corsets, which had already begun to look like what we would later call girdles, slid down the body and shifted from shaping the waist to shaping the hips. Most corsets no longer incorporated a bust area at all, meaning women had to rely on newfangled bras instead. The idea of shapewear being about *reducing* curves, as opposed to creating or exaggerating them (an idea that continues to the present day), appeared during this time as well.

After World War II, famed fashion designer Christian Dior debuted his New Look, which featured both hip pads and a waist cincher, bringing back the iconic hourglass silhouette. Dior's New Look also led to a brief revival of the corset, now called a *guepiere*, merry widow, waspie, or corselet. Women who didn't want quite as exaggerated a waist wore girdles instead. Girdles shaped the body and had the added benefit of giving a way to hold up stockings.

It wasn't until the mod era of the 1960s, when hemlines rose and led to the invention of pantyhose, that girdles more or less disappeared for good. The idea of having a naturally firm body, without the need for external aids, became popular and it was seen as old-fashioned to rely on heavy, firm shapewear underneath your clothing.

While shapewear hasn't disappeared, it's far more flexible and less structured than in decades past. Tubular garments, often knit without seams and meant to blend invisibly with the skin (to ideally look like you're not wearing any shapewear at all when dressed), are the norm. The new shapewear is about subtly influencing the figure you have, not creating a new figure outright. Fibers like spandex and nylon have also made shapewear more bendable and durable than ever before (see page 50 for more about lingerie fibers). Yet the shapewear of previous generations hasn't disappeared altogether. Corsets are still worn by a growing niche of enthusiasts, and bustiers and merry widows are still popular choices for formal events, like weddings. The big difference now is that we have more options than ever before as well as the privilege of choosing—and wearing—what we love.

How to Shop for Shapewear

Life is about feeling comfortable and beautiful in your skin, not forcing yourself to wear things you hate. I'm not here to convince anyone they have to wear shapewear, so if this section isn't for you, feel free to skip ahead. But if you're wondering how to choose sensible, safe, and, dare I say, enjoyable shapewear, then keep reading!

- **Don't buy shapewear that's too small.** I don't have many rules in this book, but this is one, and I'm afraid I really do have to insist. Many people buy shapewear a size too small because they believe tighter shapewear is more effective shapewear. That is not true. Apart from the comfort factor, too-tight shapewear can result in nerve damage, digestive issues, and even skin infections. It's not worth it! Always start by trying the size suggested for your measurements on the size chart. For most brands, this will mean knowing your waist and hip measurements (see page 53 if you're not sure how to take these). If you try a brand and it happens to run a little larger than expected, then by all means, try a smaller size. But please don't suffer or even potentially injure yourself by wearing shapewear that's too tight. If you want more shaping power, keep in mind that shapewear has several different strengths—light, medium, firm, and extra firm. If you want more of a shaping effect, considering going up a strength level before going down a size.

- **Focus on one area at a time**. While all-in-one shapers and slips are efficient, especially if you don't want to purchase multiple pieces or only want light smoothing, they're not as effective as shapewear that focuses on one specific area of the body. Prioritize the areas you want to shape and then purchase shapewear made for those exact places.

- **Expect smoothing, not slimming.** Most shapewear today won't cause dramatic changes in the way you look, but it can help give you a smooth line under clothing, especially for figure-hugging garments. Be wary of shapewear that promises dramatic effects

BONUS TIP

If your breasts are uneven by a cup size or more, fit your bra or shapewear to the larger breast and use a *cookie* or pad to fill out the cup for the smaller breast. These are usually sold in pairs and may be made of foam, gel, or silicone. Most cookies are sold in a single size (one size fits all), but some are sold by cup size (such as A/B or C/D) or as S, M, L, or XL. As with any lingerie item, reference the size chart of the brand you're interested in before buying.

like weight loss. Usually, those claims are either outright false or a side effect of losing water weight—which could leave you dangerously dehydrated!

- **Consider vintage-inspired shapewear.** Yes, I'm talking about girdles, which provide maximum shaping and body contouring, especially for retro-style fashions. There are still companies that specialize in making the kind of lingerie your grandparents used to wear. Key search terms include *corselette, open bottom girdle, longline girdle, panty girdle, waist cincher, waist nipper, waspie,* and *body briefer.*

- **Be patient.** As with everything lingerie related, remember it may take a few tries before you find the brand or style that's perfect for you. Every company is different, and experimentation is the norm, not the exception. If at all possible, try going to a well-stocked department store or lingerie boutique. There's just no substitute for trying on things in person.

Types of Shapewear

You're probably already familiar with some of the most popular types of shapewear, like control slips and shaping panties, but I think it's important to know the full range of what's available. After all, you never know when you might discover a new favorite!

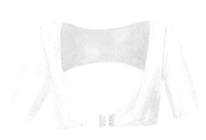

Arm Shapers

Arm shapers have fallen slightly out of favor in recent years, but they're worth a mention precisely because they're so specific. Also known as compression sleeves and slimming sleeves, arm shapers sculpt the arms from the shoulders down. Apart from the toning effects, many people even report improved posture from arm shapers, which serve as a reminder to keep their shoulders back. Arm shapers are typically available in elbow-length, three-quarter, and full-length (to the wrist) styles.

Bodysuits/Body Briefers

Bodysuits look like leotards or one-piece bathing suits. They're excellent for smoothing the torso and abdomen, and some even offer additional support and shaping to the rear and bust. While many bodysuits come with a built-in bra for maximum one-stop shopping, some bodysuits now give you the option of wearing your own bra—an ideal option for the more fuller-busted who may find the typical built-in bra to be inadequate. Some body briefers even come with longer legs (shorts or pants length) to help shape and smooth the thighs.

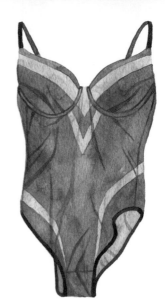

Bustiers

We already covered bustiers in on page 27, but they can also be shapewear. Bustiers were incredibly popular for formalwear during the 1950s as their long waistlines helped support and lift the bust in the strapless and low-backed evening gowns of the day. Bustiers are usually bra-sized and offer torso and waist shaping in addition to breast support. Because of this, bustiers are a popular undergarment choice for brides.

Control Briefs/Shaping Panties

Control briefs are like a bodysuit without the top portion. Shaping underwear is perfect for giving a smooth line to the low waist and pelvis, as well as lifting and sculpting the bottom. Almost all control briefs are either high-waisted (to the navel) or very high-waisted (to the ribs) for maximum shaping. Some styles even have clips or snaps to attach the shaping panty to your favorite bra. Very high-waisted styles give the most coverage and help ensure a smooth line from the bra band to the hip. If briefs aren't your style, consider a high-waisted shaping thong, which will have a shaping panel for the waist and tummy, but offer no shaping to the bottom, of course!

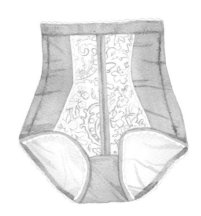

Leg Shapers/Shaping Leggings/
Shaping Shorts/Thigh Shapers

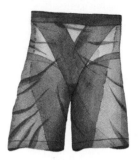

Leg shapers and shaping shorts are like bike shorts and leggings on steroids. Some people even wear their shaping shorts to the gym, though I wouldn't recommend it! Shaping shorts focus on the lower area of the body, specifically targeting the hips, rear, and thighs. Leg shapers extend from the thighs to sculpt the knees, calves, and lower legs as well. High-waisted versions of leg shapers, which rise above the navel and extend toward the rib cage, also smooth the stomach. Many present-day shapewear companies sell opaque leg shapers as everyday leggings so that you can have the support of shapewear combined with the comfort of loungewear.

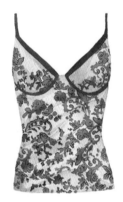

Shaping Camisoles

A body briefer without a bottom, a shaping camisole smooths the upper body, often focusing on the back, ribs, underarms, and stomach for a sleeker look. Many people like to layer shaping camisoles under thin blouses or T-shirts, as they not only sculpt the torso but also help to hide bra lines, which is especially useful for seamed or cut-and-sew bras.

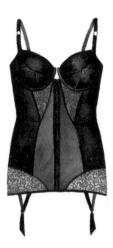

Shaping Slips/Corselettes/Shaping Dresses

Extremely popular between the 1930s and 1950s, a shaping slip is an all-in-one garment that combines a bra or camisole top with a girdle bottom. Shaping half-slips lack the upper body portion and usually start at the waist and end right above or just at the knees. Like body briefers, shaping dresses are a full body-sculpting option, smoothing the torso, waist, thighs, hips, and rear. Some shaping dresses include built-in bras as well, although wearing your own bra is an increasingly popular option.

Waist Cinchers/Waspies/Fajas

Like the bustier, the waist cincher is a contemporary equivalent to the corset, but focuses exclusively on the waist by nipping it in from the sides and flattening the torso from the front. Waist cinchers usually begin right under the bra band area and end below the waist, near the high hip. The most extreme waist cinchers are called *fajas*. Made from latex, with the ability to take in the waist by at least a couple inches, they're not for the faint of heart. Some people choose to wear their waist cinchers as belts, especially styles made with beautiful laces, prints, and fabrics.

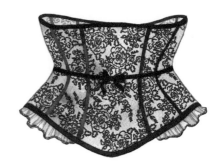

Nonshapewear Alternatives

If you've tried shapewear and it just isn't for you, take a look at one of these not-shapewear-but-still-smoothing options.

Bike Shorts

Regular microfiber bike shorts can assist with giving a smooth line under skirts and dresses without the potentially uncomfortable constriction of shapewear shorts.

Full-Cut Briefs

Covered in more detail on page 48, full-cut briefs lightly skim over the belly, hips, and rear and help to prevent panty lines.

Slips

Full-length slips help skirts and dresses hang more smoothly by lightly skimming over the body. They also blur bra and panty lines. Finally, some slips are incredibly glamorous, especially if you happen to purchase a vintage one (see page 101 for my top vintage-lingerie buying tips).

Thigh Bands

Think of a thigh band as the lace top to a thigh-high stocking . . . only without the stocking. Thigh bands help prevent chafing and are especially useful for people who dislike the extra coverage of either bike shorts or shaping shorts.

CORSETS

Corsets are fascinating undergarments, both as historical artifacts and as incredible examples of lingerie engineering. As mentioned earlier in this chapter, corsets are the precursors to today's shapewear, and their influence on what many see as an "ideal" feminine silhouette persists into the present.

Broadly speaking, a corset is a rigid, structured undergarment made of multiple nonstretch panels; flexible steel or plastic boning; back laces lined with metal rings, or grommets; and, in most cases, a metal loop-and-stud front closure called a busk (although some corsets close with a zipper and some corsets have no front closure at all). "Corsets" made with predominantly stretch fabrics or with hook-and-eye closures (such as those you'd find on the back of a bra) aren't true corsets; they are usually some variation of a waist cincher, girdle, or bustier.

Corsets work by shaping the body through carefully and specifically applied pressure to the torso, especially the waist. Some people believe corsets are inherently painful or harmful, and a poor-quality corset certainly can be. However, regular corset wearers describe a well-made corset as feeling like a firm hug. A corset should never hurt. If it does, it's either laced too tightly (loosen your laces and slow down!), the wrong shape for your body, or the wrong size.

Speaking of sizing, because a corset's shaping power is focused primarily on the waist, corsets are always sized by one's waist measurement in either inches or centimeters. Real corsets never use sizing like small, medium, and large, nor do they use dress sizes. Most corset makers recommend purchasing a corset about four inches smaller than your natural waist (for example: if your waist naturally measures thirty inches, your corset should be twenty-six inches). Plus-sized people or those with a high waist-hip difference may be able to lace down even tighter, to six inches below their natural waist measurement or more. Because corsets are nonstretch garments, the lacing at the back is what allows the corset to be loosened and tightened to fit the body.

Corsets come in two major categories: overbust and underbust. Overbust corsets cover the breasts, often giving enough support to replace a bra. Underbust corsets start below the bustline, usually in the bra band area, but sometimes lower on the ribs, and are ideal for both first-time corset wearers and those who enjoy wearing corsets every day. Generally speaking, underbust corsets are easier to order, wear, and pair with other garments. Within the two broad categories of overbust and underbust are a number of corset subtypes. The most popular styles include Edwardian, Victorian, sweetheart, pointed underbust, ribbon, plunge, and demi. Common corset fabrics or weaves include coutil, satin, brocade, twill, dupioni (silk), mesh, and taffeta.

Because corsets are incredibly complex garments, and because all corsets are handmade by skilled workers, they tend to be more expensive than people expect. Even a good-quality budget-friendly corset costs between $75 and $100. Corsets less than $50 are usually little more than decorative tubes and may even be dangerous to wear—basically, I don't recommend them. For a high-quality, off-the-rack corset (that is, not made-to-measure), you can expect to pay between $125 and $250. Around the $300 mark, you can commission a custom creation from a highly skilled corset maker who can design the beautiful corset of your dreams. There truly is no upper limit to corsetry; the most expensive and detailed corsets from the world's very best corsetieres can easily run into the thousands of dollars. If you're ready to take the leap into custom corsets, read "How to Buy Custom Lingerie" on page 103 for more information on the process.

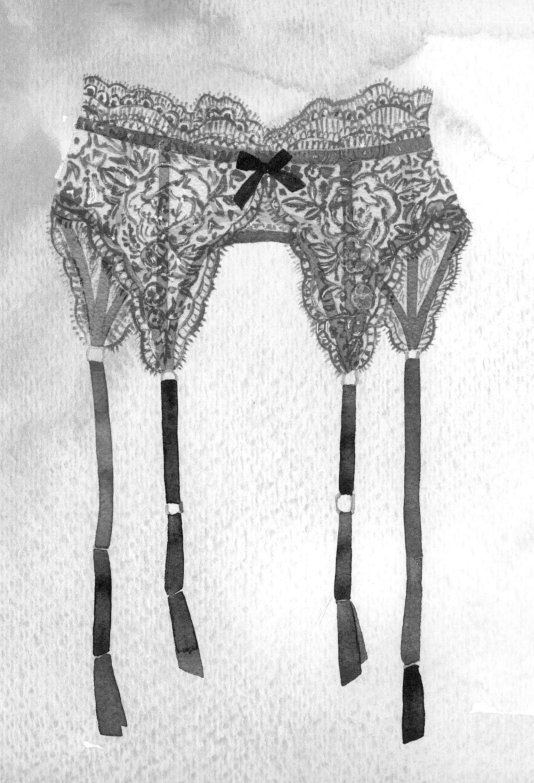

CHAPTER 4

HOSIERY

W hen I first became interested in lingerie, I started out by trying lots of different tights and stockings. Tights and pantyhose are often seen as basic, almost throwaway accessories, but they're an easy and inexpensive way to add style to any outfit. While a high-quality bra or robe can easily cost $100 or more, an elegant, well-made, fashionable pair of tights is a mere fraction of that. Hosiery is the perfect way to change your look and dip a toe into the world of lingerie.

In addition to being fashionable, hosiery can give an outfit a more polished look. Growing up in the South, tights and pantyhose were considered essential for many outfits and an outright necessity for a variety of occasions. Even today, pantyhose are often considered a part of a well-put-together ensemble, especially in the workplace or for solemn occasions.

Hosiery technically includes everything worn on the feet and legs—from socks to leggings to legwarmers, as well as the more traditional stockings, tights, pantyhose, and thigh highs. However, we'll focus exclusively on these last four items for this chapter.

A Brief History of Hosiery

Much like the first bra, it's impossible to know exactly who invented the first pair of socks or stockings. Knitted socks made between AD 250 and 420 have been discovered in Egypt, but those probably aren't the very *first* socks. The closest equivalent to modern-day hosiery likely had its origins in fourteenth-century Europe. Men wore *hose* (tights) that covered the body from waist to foot. (These eventually became pants.) Women, on the other hand, with their longer skirts, wore stockings. These ended around the knee and were held up with ribbon or fabric garters.

Early tights were made of tightly woven wool stitched together in the shape of the leg. It wasn't until the sixteenth century that knit hosiery became popular, a change that roughly coincided with the invention of the knitting machine. The knitting machine allowed stockings to be made faster and with higher quality and consistency. In addition to cotton and wool, silk—a highly breathable luxury fiber—was a popular choice for stockings, especially among royalty and the aristocracy.

Hosiery for women remained much the same for the next several centuries: stockings, that rose slightly above the knee, held up by garters. The modern-day bridal garter, traditionally worn for accessory rather than function by brides on their wedding day, is the last remnant of this former wardrobe staple.

Eventually, these individual leg garters were replaced by garter straps attached to corsets (see page 66 for more information on the corset). However, as corsets fell out of favor in the early twentieth century, garter belts rose to prominence. The shorter hemlines of the 1920s meant stockings now needed to come up somewhat higher on the leg than just above the knee.

The next major development in hosiery didn't happen until 1939—the invention of nylon. Once on the market, nylon quickly surpassed silk, cotton, rayon, and wool as the preferred stocking material because it was inexpensive, durable, and incredibly sheer. DuPont, the inventors of nylon, sold sixty-four million pairs of nylon stockings that very first year!

However, as with corsets and bras, war disrupted our lingerie story. During World War II, nylon production shifted toward military uses, such as parachutes and tents, and nylon stockings became incredibly scarce. Because bare legs simply weren't the thing to do at the time, women took to staining their legs with walnut juice or gravy and drawing a seam along the back of the leg to mimic the look of stockings.

After the war, stocking production ramped up again, but it wouldn't be long before that iconic seamed look was replaced by another type of hosiery altogether: pantyhose. Invented in 1959, pantyhose combined stockings with an attached panty, eliminating the need for a separate garter belt or girdle and immediately cutting down on the number of layers a woman was required to wear to look "presentable."

The higher hemlines and miniskirts of the 1960s (along with the concurrent invention of spandex) sealed pantyhose's fate as the heir to nylon stockings. Ever since then, pantyhose have outsold stockings.

BONUS TIP

If it's hard to make time for hand washing, you can wash your hosiery, bras, and other items of lingerie while you're in the shower.

Though nylon never lost its spot as the most popular hosiery fiber, a select number of brands still make stockings in silk, wool, or cotton, offering a wide range of options, especially for people who prefer or can only wear natural fibers. Nowadays, people are just as likely to go bare-legged as they are to wear hosiery, but stockings, tights, and pantyhose still offer a fun and financially accessible way to dress up an outfit or express your personal style. Whether you love that sheer look, lashings of lace, or vivid multicolored prints, there's hosiery out there for you!

Types of Hosiery

What's the difference between thigh highs and stockings? Or between pantyhose or tights? Keep reading for a quick primer on the most popular types of hosiery!

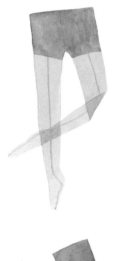

Pantyhose

Pantyhose are a sheer, all-in-one style featuring a panty attached to hosiery legs. Pantyhose are meant to replace the more outmoded combination of stockings with a girdle or garter belt. Pantyhose may be sheer all over ("sheer to waist") or may have an opaque or reinforced panty section, as in the case of control-top or shaping pantyhose. Pantyhose are typified by their sheerness (low denier; see page 74), and while they are most often worn in a color approximating the wearer's natural skin tone, they may also be another neutral color such as black. Pantyhose often provide an airbrushed effect to the legs, evening out the skin and blurring scars, bruises, veins, and blemishes.

Stockings

Stockings are a type of hosiery that extend to the upper thigh. If the stockings end at the knee, they are called *knee highs*. Modern-day stockings are almost always made of nylon, and their distinguishing feature is that they need a garter belt or leg garters to keep them up. Contemporary stockings tend to be knit into a seamless style, often with a reinforced heel and/or toe. However, fully fashioned stockings (vintage-style stockings, which are first knit flat and then sewn up the back in the shape of the leg) are still produced by a handful of factories.

Thigh Highs

Thigh highs are stockings that don't require leg garters or a garter belt to stay up (hence their other name, *stay-up stockings* or *holdups*). Elastic or silicone bands in the welt of the stocking help the stocking grip the leg and stay high on its own. Thigh highs are a relatively recent invention, but many find them to be easier to wear and more versatile than stockings.

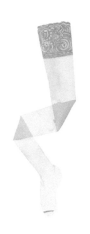

Tights

Tights fit tightly to the body (hence the name) and are essentially opaque pantyhose. Like pantyhose, they cover the entire lower body from the waist down, including the feet. Tights without the foot portion are called *leggings*. Unlike pantyhose, which are often sheer and meant to mimic skin, tights come in a wide range of colors, patterns, fabrics, and designs, including electric neons, delicate lace, insulating wool, and so on. Pantyhose made of mesh, like fishnets, are usually called tights as well. In the U.K., the word "tights" is used for both sheer pantyhose and more opaque/patterned hosiery.

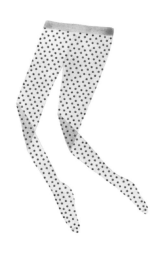

Helpful Hosiery Terminology

As with other facets of the lingerie industry, hosiery has an extensive and unique vocabulary all its own. When you're ready to shop, consult this list so you know what terms to use to find that perfect pair of pantyhose, stockings, thigh highs, or tights.

COMPRESSION STOCKINGS

Compression stockings are a special kind of hosiery meant to apply graduated pressure, or compression, to the leg. Compression stockings help improve blood flow from the legs to the heart and are especially useful during pregnancy, after surgery, or for people in occupations that require extensive periods of standing or sitting. Compression hose are also good for people with medical conditions that impair circulation, such as varicose veins or diabetes. Because compression stockings are a medical device, please consult your doctor to learn if compression stockings are a good idea for you.

Control Top

Control-top hosiery is a shapewear/pantyhose hybrid style, with the panty portion of the hosiery giving significant figure shaping (or *control* to the waist, hips, bottom, upper thighs, or some combination thereof). Control-top tights and pantyhose are meant to prevent the need to wear two separate undergarments—shapewear and pantyhose.

Denier

Denier refers to the thickness (or sheerness, depending on your perspective) of hosiery. A lower denier number indicates greater sheerness, while a higher denier number indicates a more opaque stocking. A lower denier also means a more delicate or easy-to-tear stocking. Deniers below 10 are termed ultra sheer and are best reserved for special occasions. Deniers of 10, 15, or 20 are considered sheer and are good for everyday wear. Deniers between the 30 to 40 mark are considered semiopaque, while deniers above 50 are opaque to the degree that you can't see the leg through the fabric. Superhigh deniers, 100 or above, are ideal for cold weather, as they're very thick and insulating.

Finish

Hosiery finish is a continuum from shiny to matte. A shiny finish (also known as gloss, glimmer, luster, shine, or sheen) is bright and sparkling, reflecting light in a way many find aesthetically pleasing (think of it as giving the look of freshly oiled legs). Matte or flat hosiery has a duller finish that doesn't reflect light and is perfect for more serious occasions.

Gusset

The gusset is an extra bit of fabric usually sewn onto the crotch seam in pantyhose and tights. The gusset adds comfort and durability to a high-stress part of the garment (where the legs divide). If made of cotton, or a similar fabric with moisture-wicking capabilities, it enhances breathability for the genital area.

Ladder

A ladder is a tear in the hosiery. It occurs when the knit yarn comes undone or is ripped. Ladders look like a long, vertical hole with a series of horizontal fibers running across it, thus the term. If you find your stockings ladder often, look for hosiery described as *run resistant.*

Toe

The toe of your hosiery can be sheer, reinforced, shadow, or open. A sandalfoot or invisible toe has no reinforcement and is sheer nylon all along the foot. A reinforced toe has thicker knit nylon at the toe to help prevent runs; this thicker knit also results in a more opaque toe (and also heel, if that area is reinforced as well). A shadow toe is in between a sandalfoot and reinforced toe—not as sheer as the sandalfoot, but also not as thick as the traditional reinforced toe. Open toe or toeless hosiery ends just before the toes, leaving them free and exposed.

Welt

Welt is a term specific to stockings and thigh highs. It usually refers to the upper portion of the stocking, which is thicker and more opaque than the rest of the leg. The welt is where you attach the garter grips if you're wearing stockings that require garters. The welt is also where silicone bands or elastic would be placed if you're wearing thigh highs. Finally, the welt is what you'll want to grab to pull on your stockings so as to avoid tearing the more delicate leg.

Hosiery Advice

Here are a few tips to keep in mind as you shop for hosiery.

- Always make sure your legs and feet are well moisturized before putting on your hosiery. Be sure to trim any hangnails or rough nail edges. Also file down or exfoliate any rough skin. A quick slathering of baby oil or lotion on your legs can also help prevent runs and ladders. And if you shave your legs regularly, make sure there's no new stubble before pulling on your stockings.

- The one exception to the moisturizing rule? Thigh highs! Lotion or oil will prevent the silicone bands on your welts from gripping the skin, which will make your thigh highs fall down. Avoid any moisturizers on your upper thighs if you plan to wear stay-ups. Also note that thigh highs with a wide welt tend to stay up better than thigh highs with a narrow one.

- If it's going to be a while until you put your shoes on after putting on your hosiery, slip on a pair of socks or slippers to avoid snags or stubbing your toe (stockings can be slippery!).

- If you have rough hands, long fingernails, or are just generally clumsy (like me!), invest in a pair of hosiery gloves. These can be purchased from specialty hosiery retailers or lingerie boutiques, but if you don't have one of those near you, a simple pair of plain knit gloves will do. Ideally, you want to keep your fingers from snagging those delicate, finely woven yarns and potentially laddering or tearing your tights.

- When putting on your stockings, first remove all jewelry and put on your hosiery gloves, if you have them. After gathering your hosiery in your hand, start at the toes and ankle and gradually work the hosiery up your leg. Avoid pulling hosiery up by the waistband alone. Think of it as unrolling a scroll: you wouldn't start in the middle; instead you'd begin at one end and slowly work your way to the other.

- If your hosiery does happen to run or tear, a little hairspray on the spot or a dab of clear nail polish will stop the run from spreading. If using nail polish, you'll want to lightly paint or dot the edges of the run. If using hairspray, lightly spray all over the tear, being careful not to get hairspray on your clothes or shoes.

- Ready to get fancy? Look for stockings with *clocking*, a type of decoration along the ankles and calves; *fancy-heeled stockings*, stockings with decorative details such as an outlined heel; or embellished, embroidered, lacy, or patterned stockings.

- Never, *ever* throw your stockings in the dryer, as this will destroy them. Always hand wash your hosiery, preferably with a lingerie or delicates wash, and hang them to dry away from any direct heat sources.

HOW TO BUY A GARTER BELT

Garter belts can be a fun and exciting item, and if you're unable to wear pantyhose or tights, also a practical one. If you're interested in a good daily garter belt (the kind that can actually hold up to walking and all-day wear), keep the following points in mind.

- A quality garter belt should have at least six straps. While many garter belts sold in stores have only four, this is not enough to keep your stockings in place. Three garter straps on each leg secure the stocking on the front, back, and outside of the leg. This keeps the hosiery from twisting around the thigh, which reduces stress on the stocking and helps prevent laddering and runs. In addition, assuming you don't have a metal allergy, the garter clips should be metal, not plastic. Metal clips are more durable, comfortable, and easier to fasten than plastic.

- The belt portion of your garter belt should be fairly wide, at least the width of the palm of your hand or if not more. A wide garter belt provides a good anchor, especially when worn at the natural waist. High-quality garter belts are sized by your waist measurement (where your body naturally creases if you bend to the side; see page 53 if you're unsure how to measure your waist).

- While some garter belts are a slip-on style, I recommend choosing one with hook-and-eye closures at the back (like a bra). Hooks and eyes allow for maximum security and adjustability. Delicate or strappy garter belts are cute, but not as effective for holding up your stockings.

- A high-quality garter belt is made of durable materials like satin, power mesh, or nonstretch lace. Overly stretchy, thin, or flimsy materials, while appropriate for the boudoir, can lose shape quickly and aren't strong enough for long-term wear. Look for plain, smooth materials with minimal ornamentation (ruffles, bows, etc.) so that your garter belt doesn't show through your clothing.

Finally, to answer the age-old question, if you plan on wearing your garter belt out and about, make sure you wear your underwear on top of the garter straps. Even if that's not the way it's shown in the magazines, it's much more comfortable, convenient, and practical!

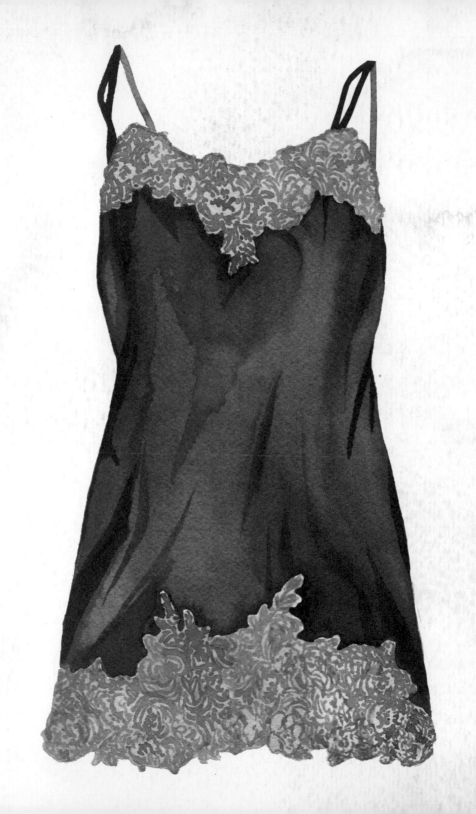

CHAPTER 5

LOUNGEWEAR

L ingerie is ultimately a treat for yourself. Nowhere is this more evident than in loungewear. While the concept of having lingerie specifically to wear at home may seem frivolous and pointless at first glance, it's actually a way of taking care of yourself in the place you spend the most time—at home, among family and friends. Home is where comfort matters most; after all, where can you feel relaxed if not in your own residence?

Loungewear is also an incredibly economical purchase, in terms of cost per wear. A high-quality robe or pair of pajamas can last for years, worn day after day, month after month, season after season. The cost per wear can literally be counted in pennies over time. No other type of lingerie offers such value, such bang for your buck. And now that casual, comfortable loungewear is so popular, there are an astonishing number of options to choose from—whether your style is yoga pants and hoodies or glamorous, vintage-inspired robes.

A Brief History of Loungewear

The idea of loungewear, or lingerie that exists solely to wear around the house, appeared in Western fashion during the Rococo era (1650–1800). However, please note that Europeans did not invent loungewear; for example, robes were worn in Japan long before this period! In seventeenth century Europe, the idea of choosing clothing purely for comfort's sake was a novel one. Keeping warm, showing one's wealth, and conforming to regional trends and laws were all considered more important than comfort.

The negligee, one of the first items of European-style loungewear, made its appearance during the reign of France's Louis XIV (1643–1715). The negligee was worn specifically during the morning *toilette* (a sort of dressing ceremony that involved getting ready for the day) and was worn only at home.

While the concept of nightwear, or clothes to wear to bed, closely overlaps with loungewear, what distinguishes loungewear from nightwear is that the former is meant to be worn outside of the bed itself—unlike nightwear (which is also known by the name sleepwear).

In the eighteenth century, dressing gowns or wrapping gowns, came into vogue. What stands out about the dressing gown is its informality, especially for women. These gowns were loose, with little to no definition around the waist, and offered aristocratic, upper-class women (the only women who had real leisure time in this era, as well as the money to spend on clothes worn only at home) a break from the stays, petticoats, and heavy gowns of daily dress.

While in her dressing gown, a woman could complete her morning rituals of bathing, hairdressing, entertaining friends, writing letters, working on needlework, eating breakfast, and choosing the outfit or activities for the day. Furthermore, in an era where wealthy women might change outfits multiple times per day, a dressing gown gave them the opportunity to recline and relax between social events. Dressing gowns also protected equally lavish undergarments, like stays and petticoats, from stray cosmetics or hair powder while women were dressing.

By the nineteenth century, dressing gowns had trickled down from the upper classes into the middle and lower classes. They also became more ornate and more fitted to the figure. The most expensive dressing gowns were made from silk (often expensively embroidered kimono silks or lushly quilted silk satins) and were often trimmed in feathers or lace. Less-expensive gowns might be made from fabrics like calico or chintz.

Pajamas, one of the most famous items of loungewear, were everyday wear in India, but not introduced to Europeans until the seventeenth century (the word *pajamas* or *pyjamas* was adopted into English from the Hindi or Hindustani language, with the word originating from the Persian language). Adopted by the British as loungewear, pajamas became immensely popular for men in the Victorian era, around the late nineteenth century. However, it wasn't until the 1920s and 1930s that pajamas were seen as acceptable attire for women. At first, pajamas were worn solely as beachwear, as they were easy to slip on over a bathing suit for warmth or modesty's sake. Gradually, it became acceptable to wear them inside the home as well, as lounging pajamas (a useful item for seeing guests) or as nightwear.

Throughout the early twentieth century, dressing gowns remained popular, especially for wearing over a nightgown, but they began to transform into the shorter, more abbreviated shapes we recognize now: the bathrobe, peignoir, and bed jacket. The nightgown also underwent a metamorphosis during this time, changing from the shapeless white linen and cotton of previous centuries to colorful nylon, silk, and rayon garments in figure-hugging shapes. In particular, the nightgowns of the 1930s and 1940s imitated popular evening-gown silhouettes of the era and featured bias cuts, V-necks, halter necks, and low and open backs. While the ankle-length nightgown still exists, our shorter, more modern babydolls, chemises, and negligees all derive from this early-twentieth-century transformation of the nightgown.

Today, loungewear can double as outerwear. People wear pajamas, nightgowns, chemises, and bed jackets outside the home in increasingly bold ensembles. And in an era where people are likely to spend their weekends entertaining at home or binge-watching their favorite shows, comfortable loungewear has more utility and purpose than ever before.

Modern-day loungewear also takes a cue from athletic wear. Sweatpants, yoga pants, sweatshirts, tank tops, fleece hoodies, and jersey shorts are all just as good for lounging around the house as they are for running errands or hitting the gym.

Casual, even unisex, loungewear, unimaginable in centuries past, is now common. No longer limited exclusively to the wealthy, today people can feel free to wear their loungewear wherever, and however they like.

BONUS TIP

To maximize your options, look for items that can do double duty as both loungewear and outerwear—for example: tunics, sweatshirts, camisoles, track pants, and leggings.

Types of Loungewear & Sleepwear

From babydolls and bed jackets to caftans and camisoles, the world of loungewear is an exciting one to explore. Let's move beyond the bathrobe and discuss your options!

Babydolls

A babydoll is a short, high-waisted nightgown that hangs loosely from the bustline or even directly from the shoulders. Babydolls almost always end above the knee. They're a beautiful, body-skimming alternative to chemises for people who may feel a little self-conscious about their tummies, thighs, or hips, and the loose cut makes them a highly size-flexible option.

Bed Jackets

A bed jacket is a short (usually not more than waist or hip length), sleeved jacket worn over a nightgown, chemise, peignoir, or similar item. Bed jackets were popular in the early to mid-twentieth century, as they allowed the wearer to sit up in bed and have breakfast while remaining warm and covered (the bed jacket ended where the bedcovers began). Bed jackets are less popular today, but more versatile. Many can be styled as light jackets or capelets and worn as outerwear.

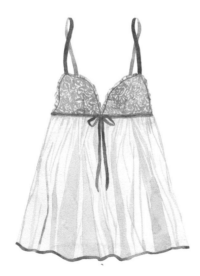

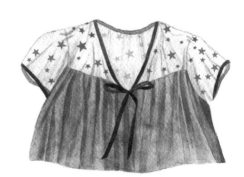

Caftans

A caftan is an unstructured, ankle-length, long-sleeved tunic. Caftans are thousands of years old and originated in the Middle East, specifically Mesopotamia, though the word is Persian. Nowadays, loosely fitting, billowing caftans are not only worn around the home, they also make a glamorous poolside lounging option, especially as a swimsuit cover-up.

Camisoles

A camisole is a sleeveless top, usually characterized by thin, bra-style straps. Victorian corset covers are the predecessors of the modern-day camisole. Camisoles are shorter than chemises, usually ending around the waist or high hip; longer than that and a camisole becomes a chemise or nightgown. Camisoles make wonderful layering pieces, especially for a lingerie-as-outerwear look or to cover up a lacy or seamed bra. (I also like wearing them under sweaters in the winter!)

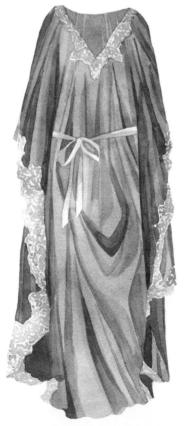

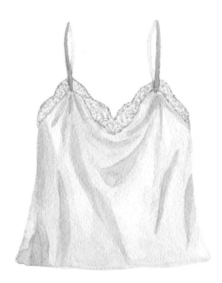

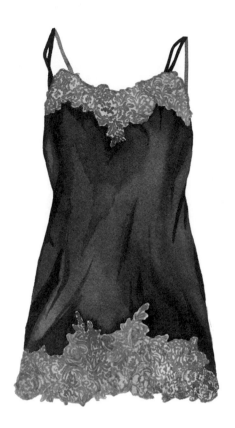

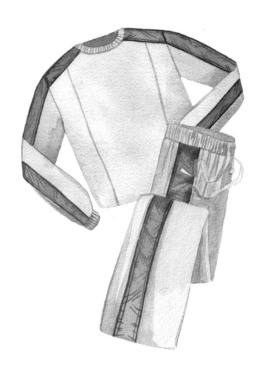

Chemises

A chemise is a short, slightly fitted gown similar in shape, fit, and construction to a knee-length full slip. Some people even wear their slips as chemises! Chemises can be simple or embellished and are the perfect introduction to loungewear, as they tend to be very accessible in terms of size, price, style, and color.

Lounge Sets

A lounge set is usually composed of a top and pants. Lounge sets bear a close resemblance to pajamas but tend to be styled in a way that makes them suitable for outerwear as well (for example, a yoga pant and hoodie set or a track suit).

Nightgowns

A nightgown is a dress-like type of sleepwear, often extending below the knees. Nightgowns may be loose and unstructured or cut on the bias and fitted. Nightgowns may also be either sleeved or sleeveless and made with any type of neckline (V-neck, halter neck, off the shoulder, etc.) or back (low back, strappy, sheer back, etc.). Nightgowns always extend below the waist and may reach the floor. Both modern-day chemises and babydolls have their origins in nightgowns.

Nightshirts

A nightshirt is a long, pajama-style top, meant to be worn on its own and ending at the mid-thigh or knees. Simple nightshirts are usually buttonless and can be slipped on over the head; they may also be called tunics.

Pajamas

Pajamas are two-piece garments composed of a top paired with shorts or pants bottoms. Traditional pajamas consist of a long-sleeved, button-up jacket paired with long pants. In contrast, contemporary pajamas can feature a camisole, T-shirt, or short-sleeved button-up style top combined with either shorts or pants for the bottom.

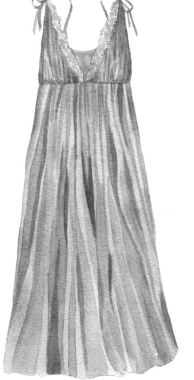

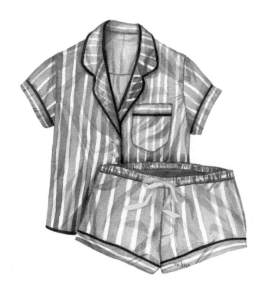

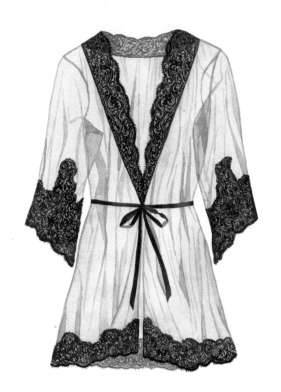
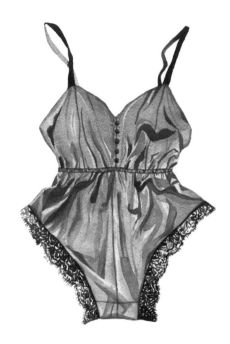

Robes

A robe is a loose-fitting, sleeved garment that usually ties or wraps in the front. Robes can be elaborate and luxurious (such as those made from embroidered satin or silk velvet) or they can be simple and practical (such as those made from terry cloth or jersey). Robes may be either long or short, but they always extend past the waist. Like chemises, robes are another excellent introductory item, as their loose construction and wide range of styles mean almost everyone can find a robe they like.

Teddies

A teddy, also known as a romper, is a garment made of a top and shorts (or knickers) sewn together. While the top is usually in the camisole style, it may also be a T-shirt style or even long-sleeved. Fitted one-pieces with brief or thong style bottoms are called bodysuits. One-pieces that combine long pants with a top are referred to as jumpsuits or catsuits.

Loungewear Advice

Here are a few tips to keep in mind as you shop for loungewear.

- **Buy the best-quality loungewear you can afford.** Because loungewear is meant to be worn at home and because you likely spend a lot of time at home, you want your loungewear to be something you are excited about and look forward to wearing.

- **Pay close attention to the fabric composition.** Give priority to breathable, natural fibers whenever possible. (See page 50 for more information on the different kinds of fibers.) If nylon makes you sweat or polyester makes you itch, don't choose loungewear made from those materials. Similarly, pick loungewear you can easily wash and take care of at home. Most of us don't have the budget to dry clean our lingerie, so even if that floor-length silk robe with feather trim takes your breath away, remember to factor in the cost of taking care of it.

- **Think of how you plan to wear your loungewear and buy accordingly**. If you envision yourself wearing a robe while cooking breakfast, long, kimono-inspired sleeves likely aren't the best idea. Even if something is beautiful, it's no good to you if you're afraid to wear it. Buy loungewear you'll feel comfortable wearing—in every way.

FABRICS VERSUS FIBERS

Many people confuse fabrics and fibers; however, knowing the difference between the two is important when lingerie shopping. Generally speaking, a fiber is the raw or base material. For example, cotton, silk, flax (the fiber that makes linen), wool, polyester, and nylon are all types of fibers.

A fabric is the finished textile or cloth—the product of weaving, knitting, or knotting the original fiber. Popular fabrics for lingerie and loungewear include satin, charmeuse, chiffon, crepe de chine, chambray, flannel, fleece, lace, georgette, jersey, mesh, tulle, and velvet.

A descriptor like *silk satin* means the fiber content is silk (or, more likely, a silk elastane blend for stretch and durability) and the type of fabric, or weave, is satin. Always be sure to check the fiber content of the garment you're buying, especially if you have allergies or skin sensitivities. Brands are required by law to publicly share this information, usually on a tag sewn to the garment itself.

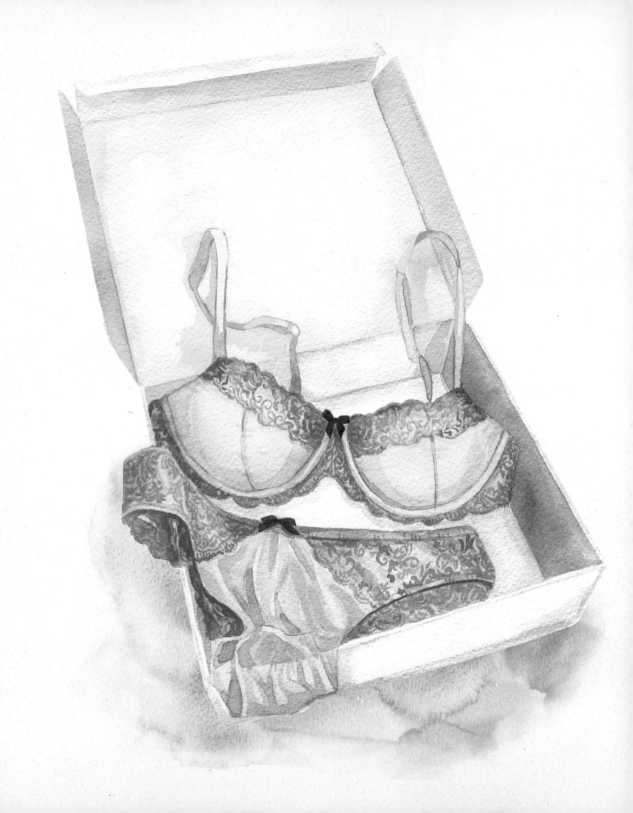

CHAPTER 6

SHOPPING

$\mathcal{N}$ow that we've covered the basics, it's time to get to the fun stuff—how to shop! For centuries, the only way to buy lingerie was to have it custom made, an expensive and time-consuming process. Today, however, we're lucky that almost anything we want is available instantly—it only requires a trip to a store, a click of the mouse, or a tap on the screen.

However, all these options also mean there's more room for error. How do you know if you're buying the best bra, pair of underwear, or waist cincher when there are so many versions available? How do you know if you're buying from the best store or the best product for your particular body? Though shopping can—and should!—be fun, it can also be stressful and anxiety inducing, especially if you're not yet comfortable buying lingerie.

More than anything, try to have a good time and enjoy the experience. Lingerie is a way of expressing your personal style, identity, and sense of self. We all deserve that. Lingerie is about pleasing yourself and treating yourself first and foremost. Because you deserve beautiful things, and you deserve to enjoy wearing them.

How to Shop for Lingerie in a Store

While online boutiques and retailers like Amazon, Etsy, and eBay have taken off, there's still nothing quite like shopping for lingerie in a brick-and-mortar store. A good boutique or department store offers services you simply can't get online: personalized attention, the ability to try before you buy, even special orders in a different color or hard-to-find size. Furthermore, a good lingerie shop—one that's local to you and you can visit regularly—can be your best ally. They want you as a long-term customer, and they want you to feel happy enough with your experience to tell a friend. Not only can a good brick-and-mortar shop help you find the perfect lingerie, it can also be a direct connection between you and your favorite brands. Stores tell lingerie companies what their customers want to see more of, whether that's a different shape, more colors, extended sizes, new fabrics, or even lower prices!

However, the experience of shopping in a store can also be very intimidating. On several occasions, I've gone to a lingerie shop, excited and ready to buy, only to be flatly ignored. Other people have had even worse experiences, from being turned away for not looking "feminine enough" to being told the store had no interest in helping people of their size. While shopping at a boutique can be a fantastic experience, it can also be stressful, and you shouldn't shop anywhere you are mistreated. Take your business to someone who appreciates it and you!

However, if you haven't visited your local lingerie store and are ready to give it a try, here are a few of my favorite shopping tips.

- **Seek out specialists**. If at all possible, go to a specialty lingerie boutique or a department store with a dedicated lingerie department and a knowledgeable sales staff. Reviews on websites like Yelp can help you find the best spots near you. Whether you're shopping at a small, locally owned store or a larger, national retail chain, you want to feel confident that you're talking to a lingerie specialist, someone who is there because they love lingerie and want to help you.

- **Call ahead**. If you're shopping for a special occasion, you're new to lingerie shopping (for example, this is your first time buying a bra), or you've recently experienced a major life-changing event (such as a mastectomy or pregnancy), it's perfectly acceptable to call the store ahead of time. You may want to make a fitting appointment, so they can set aside some time for you. You can even ask if they carry certain styles, brands, or products you're interested in. For example, if you're pregnant, ask if the shop stocks maternity bras before making a special trip. If you're nervous or anxious about visiting the store, it's okay to bring a friend, but make sure your friend is a supportive sort of person, not a judgmental one! Finally, if the store has an online presence, check it out first to get a sense of their style and what they like to carry.

- **Try to put yourself in a good, or at least neutral, frame of mind.** Have a small meal before going to shop. Wear an outfit you like and comfy shoes. If at all possible, try not to go during a time when you're struggling with strong self-doubt or low

BONUS TIP

Since bra bands stretch out over time, wear your new bras on their loosest hook. Then, as the elastic stretches, you can move to tighter hooks, preserving your bra!

self-esteem. Lingerie shopping causes enough anxiety all on its own. Be in the best mood you can be before starting.

- **Have a sense of what you want.** While the retail staff is there to help you, they can't decide your tastes for you. Are you into sporty, minimalist underwear? Do you like frills and lace? Are you just there for the basics? It's okay if you're not sure what you like yet. Simply being able to express how you want to feel is helpful too (for example, "I want to feel glamorous but comfortable"). Related to this, have a budget in mind. If you know you can't spend more than $50 on a bra, let the salesperson know so you don't fall in love with a bra that's $150.

- **Be willing to experiment.** If you wear only full-coverage T-shirt bras, give a demi or a plunge style a try. Never worn loungewear before? Slip a robe or two into the mix. It's very easy to enter a boutique and assume nothing will look right on you, but that may not be case. If you think something is pretty on the hanger, try it on your body. And, as a brief aside, please remember to keep your own underwear on when trying lingerie.

- **If it's been a while since you've been fitted, get fitted.** More than that, be open to wearing a new and different size. Everyone's bra size changes over their lifetime. You may have worn a 32D five years ago, but now you wear a 36E and that's okay. *You are not your bra size.* A bra size is just a number and a letter to help you find the best-fitting undergarments. In the same vein, remember that your size may change across brands and styles. As mentioned in chapter 1, this is totally normal and not a reflection on you or your body.

- **Try on a lot of bras.** When shopping for bras, expect to try on many styles before finding one that's right for you. Bras are finicky. Even slight variations in wire width, fabric composition, and strap placement can affect how they fit and feel on the body. That's a good thing because it means more people can find the bras they love. However, the downside is that you may have to go through a few (or a lot) before finding your perfect fit. Be patient. Everyone has to do this part. It's worth it when you find a bra you love!

- **Take a break**. If you start to feel overwhelmed or frustrated, it's totally fine to get a breath of fresh air or step out of the store. A good salesperson will understand and won't pressure you.

- **Don't buy something unless you absolutely love it**. I'm serious. If you don't feel confident and comfortable and like this is the perfect garment for you, don't buy it. Otherwise, it'll just sit in the back of your underwear drawer forever. If you do love something and feel ready to buy it, check the store's return policy first. Many stores won't allow returns of underwear for obvious reasons. Some stores have exchange-only policies, while others only offer things on final sale. Whatever the policy is, make sure you know it and agree with it before purchasing.

- **If the sales staff in a store make you uncomfortable, leave.** They don't deserve your time and money, and that's not a shop you want to patronize. Go to the stores that want your business!

How to Shop for Lingerie Online

While there are definite perks to shopping for lingerie in person, sometimes it's just not possible. Distance, time, and ease can make shopping and trying things on from the comfort of your home a better option. Thankfully, lingerie shopping online is easy and can also be a great way to explore at your own pace.

Online lingerie shopping is also ideal if you already know your size and style and are just "refilling" on basics. Additionally, online shops are great if you're looking for certain specialty products (such as metal- or elastic-free bras) that are impossible to find in stores. Finally, online shopping is perfect for hard-to-find brands or sizes. Some European brands, for example, aren't sold in any American stores, so the only way to buy them is online. And, of course, if you're a bargain hunter, online shopping is great for that as well.

One of the most important things to know when buying online is that you're purchasing from a reputable retailer. Unfortunately, it's easy for sketchy "businesses" to set up a fake online storefront and take people's money with no intention of sending the goods. Avoid being scammed by doing your research ahead of time.

Look for online reviews (lingerie blogs are great for this) or visit online forums and communities to read what other people have said about the store in which you're interested (online reviews are also great for learning about things you can't see from a computer screen . . . such as how the fabric feels to the touch or if it has any signs of poor construction). And remember: If a deal seems too good to be true, it probably is.

Here are some other helpful tips to keep in mind when shopping online.

- **Know your size and fit.** You should already know your bra size and how a bra should fit if you're buying from the internet (see page 34 for more information on how your bra should fit). Online shopping is wonderful for trying out different styles and brands, but it's easy to get overwhelmed if you don't already have an idea of what you want or like.

- **Be diligent about reading reviews.** Read reviews of brands. Read reviews of stores. And also read reviews of the products you want to buy. Many online stores have review sections, and you should read both positive and negative reviews. If a website only has positive reviews, be skeptical. No product is 100 percent perfect for 100 percent of the people 100 percent of the time. The store may be hiding or deleting negative reviews in an effort improve the ratings of a problematic product.

- **Read the return and shipping policies.** Is trackable shipping an option? What happens if your package is lost? Do they accept returns without fuss, or will you need to get their permission first? Will you get your money back or receive store credit only? Don't assume different stores will have similar policies.

- **Try it on.** Once you receive the item you ordered, try it on as soon as possible and always over your own undergarments. Be careful not to soil, stain, or otherwise mark the product—that means no deodorant stains, no perfume scents, no hairspray— nothing. Any sign of wear means the company won't be able to accept the return. That makes sense, right? You wouldn't want to wear underwear that someone has already worn and dirtied either!

- **If you know you're not keeping something**, box it up and send it back straightaway. The sooner you make your return, the better. And don't forget to leave a review of your own! The more information available, the better shopping is for everyone.

How to Give the Gift of Lingerie

One quick note before beginning this section: Lingerie is an intimate gift, no pun intended. It's not a gift for casual acquaintances or recent relationships. If you don't know the person very well and aren't completely confident they'll receive your gift of lingerie with gratitude, avoid giving them lingerie. That said, it can be a fun present for a partner or close friend. Here's some advice for how to lingerie shop for others.

- **Splurge!** Treat your giftee to an indulgence they may not otherwise buy for themselves. This isn't the time to reach for everyday knickers; try to expand your horizons—and theirs as well.

- **Avoid bra-sized items**. Bras are difficult to buy, because, as you now know, there is no consistency in sizing. Instead, consider giving items like robes, chemises, pajama sets, and caftans. Even a really great pair of bedroom slippers can be an awesome gift.

- **Consider the fabric.** You can never go wrong with high-end fabrics like cashmere and silk—unless, of course, the gift recipient is a vegan, in which case look at textiles like bamboo and linen.

- **Buy from places with customer-friendly return policies**. Put another way, avoid final-sale retailers like the plague. There are any number of reasons why your gift may not work, so purchase from a place that will let your friend easily return or exchange the item.

- **Avoid gifts that are focused on "fixing" something.** Even someone who feels very confident about their body may not enjoy a gift of shapewear. Instead, give priority to lingerie that offers an experience of luxury, relaxation, or indulgence.

BONUS TIP

Don't forget gift cards! Gift cards may have a bad reputation as being a lazy gift, but they genuinely are the best way to ensure your gift recipients can buy exactly what they want.

THE SIGNS OF HIGH-QUALITY LINGERIE

As with everything else, there's a wide range of quality available when it comes to lingerie, and some pieces are simply better than others. However, "luxury" is a popular buzzword that almost every brand uses—whether they've earned it or not—so how can you tell if the piece you want to buy is truly well-made and worth the money?

The two most important things to look at when assessing your lingerie are materials and construction. Pay attention to what's called the *hand* of the fabric, that is, how it feels to the touch. High-quality lingerie fabrics will feel smooth and soft. Low-quality fabrics will feel rough, scratchy, or stiff. Keep in mind that however a fabric feels to your hand, that feeling will be magnified on your body, so don't ignore your sense of touch.

Speaking of materials, you also want to look at the hardware on the lingerie: hooks, eyes, closures, adjusters, fasteners, and the like. Are they made of metal or plastic? Do they look flimsy or sturdy? For luxury lingerie especially, custom hardware, such as clasps or clips with the company's logo or name, are often an indicator of high quality.

Next, look closely at the construction of the undergarment. Does the design look balanced and thoughtful, or does it appear haphazard and sloppy? If there is a lace motif, embroidery, or a print on the garment, does the pattern align or match?

Then examine the stitching. Is it even and regular? Are all the seams and stitches straight? Are there any skipped stitches or loose threads? Regular, even, tight stitches are all signs of a high-quality garment that will last a while. Raw fabric edges, loose threads, puckered fabrics, and other irregularities are all signs of a lower-quality garment.

We all have different budgets, and most of us can't afford the most expensive lingerie available, but by knowing how to recognize a quality garment, you'll be able to buy the very best lingerie you can afford. You'll be able to tell the difference between what's truly high quality and what's just good advertising. And that's what is most important.

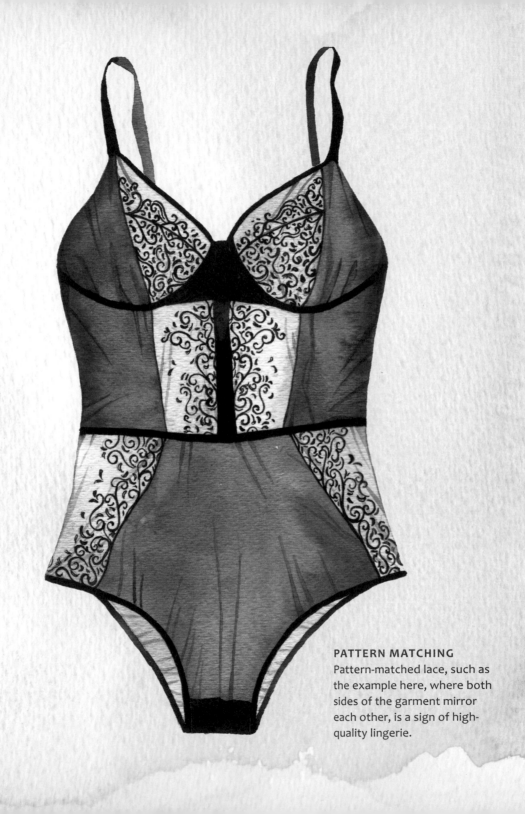

PATTERN MATCHING
Pattern-matched lace, such as the example here, where both sides of the garment mirror each other, is a sign of high-quality lingerie.

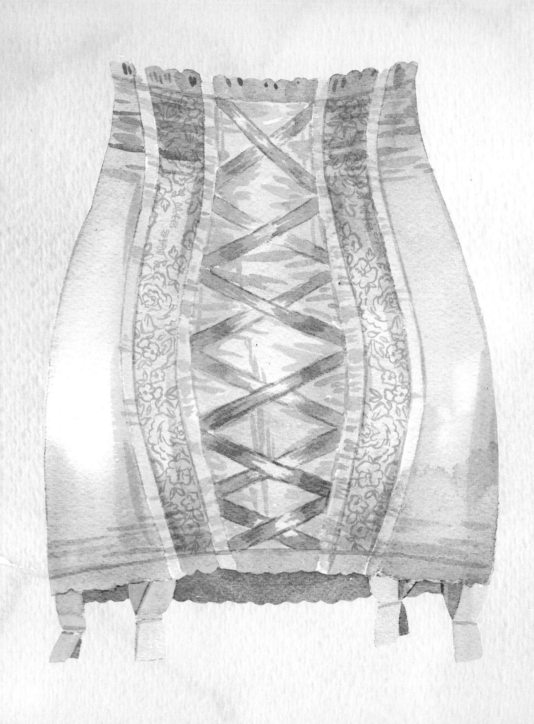

How to Shop for Vintage Lingerie

Vintage lingerie is one of my favorite things. There is a level of craftsmanship, care, and detail in vintage lingerie that simply isn't available anymore—at least not without a hefty price tag! Many of the laces and sewing techniques seen in vintage lingerie are no longer used, which means you're also owning a piece of history— something special that can never be replicated or replaced.

As a general guideline, the cutoff for calling something vintage is that it was made more than twenty years ago. A garment that's been made in modern times but has a vintage aesthetic or is adapted from a vintage pattern, is called *retro* to distinguish it from authentic vintage (some people also use the term *faux vintage*). If a garment is more than eighty years old (that is, it was last in fashion more than a few generations ago), it's considered to be an antique. Antique items tend to be both exceptionally delicate and rare, which often means they're not suitable for wearing. One notable exception, however, is antique cotton, which tends to have a much higher thread count and therefore can be much better quality than modern cotton undergarments.

An important thing to know right away is that most vintage lingerie has been worn. While most vintage sellers won't offer garments that are obviously stained, repaired, or worn out (unless these items are valuable for some other purpose, like research), if the idea of owning someone's previously worn lingerie bothers you, look for items labeled as *deadstock* or *new old stock*. These are the terms used for vintage items that have never been worn and are in their original state.

Because clothing sizes have changed significantly over the years, you always want to use your most recent measurements when determining if you should buy a vintage piece you intend to wear. A vintage size 6 is not a modern size 6, and being off by even an inch could render a garment completely unwearable.

In addition, don't be afraid to ask the seller questions, and research for yourself what authentic vintage lingerie from each era looks like. For example, the most popular lingerie colors of the 1920s were shades of blush, peach, rose pink, robin's egg blue, and mint green. If you see an item claiming to be from the 1920s, but it's hot pink or bright orange, you may want to ask the seller for clarification. Similarly, nylon wasn't invented until the mid-1930s and didn't become popular for lingerie until the 1950s. Therefore, if someone's selling a nylon nightgown or dressing gown that they claim is from the 1930s or 1940s, ask more questions so you can be sure of what you're getting.

While you're asking questions, don't forget to inquire about the condition of the item. If you are shopping online, pictures can tell you a lot, but not everything. A good seller will post photos from every angle, including detailed close-ups of any defects, stains, flaws, or repairs. At minimum, you should see photographs of the front, back, inside, and sides of the garment, as well as detail shots of any closures, buttons, zippers, or flaws.

If you have the opportunity to view the items in person, such as at an estate sale or flea market, do so, and don't be afraid to closely examine the pieces. Elastic, for example, can dry out and disintegrate over time—a terrible thing to discover once you've gotten the piece home. Also remember to check the garment for scents, keeping in mind that not all smells are easy to remove. If you've fallen in love with a garment that has a pungent or musty odor, spritzing it with a solution of vodka and water (two parts water for every one part vodka) can lift scents, as can hanging a garment outside for brief periods in the sun. If you're worried about bacteria or fabric-eating bugs, freeze your garment for up to a week, carefully folding it before placing it in a sealable plastic bag or bin (some people choose to wrap their garment in a layer of cotton or muslin cloth to absorb any condensation), and allow your garment to return to room temperature before unfolding.

Popular vintage items to purchase, especially for regular wear, include bullet bras, girdles, corselettes, knickers, garter belts, dressing gowns, robes, and petticoats. However, my favorite item of vintage lingerie is the slip. Vintage slips are far more ornate and elegant than modern slips and are perfect to wear as a nightgown, loungewear, or even a dress. Vintage slips also tend to be ridiculously inexpensive. I've seen beautiful, lace-trimmed slips online for as little as $5.

Once you purchase your vintage lingerie, proper cleaning and care is essential. Not all of the advice in chapter 7 will apply to vintage undergarments. They may be too delicate, for example, to immerse in water. Always spot test a small, inconspicuous part of the item with warm water first. You don't want that beautiful silk robe to lose all its color or even disintegrate because you submerged it without testing!

Because vintage lingerie is especially vulnerable to mold, rot, and moths, it has to be stored in special conditions as well. Avoid clamps, clips, and plastic or wire hangers, as they can stress, distort, or even tear the fabric. Also avoid plastic bags or bins as they can encourage the growth of mold. And always remember to store your vintage lingerie out of direct sunlight, as the sun can fade the colors of your delicate pieces.

How to Buy Custom Lingerie

If you have the desire (and funds) to splurge on luxury lingerie, why not consider a custom purchase? Custom lingerie gives you the opportunity to own something unique and unusual that you can't buy anywhere else. But, we can't talk about custom lingerie without discussing price. Custom undergarments can easily run into the three or four figures. However, it's worth it to own something uniquely yours that will last for years.

Lingerie designers refer to their custom services by a number of names, including *bespoke*, *made to order*, *made to measure*, *personalized*, *semi-custom*, or *couture*. The level of customization ranges from having an already existing off-the-rack pattern tweaked slightly to your specifications all the way to purchasing a truly couture set, made to order for you alone and never to be made again.

While many people take advantage of custom lingerie to address size or fit concerns, custom lingerie truly shines when you collaborate with the designer. Following are tips to create the dazzling lingerie of your dreams.

- **Have a sense of your style and taste.** If you're still figuring out what you like, now may not be the right time to order custom lingerie. In addition, consider how you plan to wear the piece. Will it be worn only at home? Is it for a special occasion? Do you want something you can wear all the time, or will it be worn only once?

- **Spend time researching designers.** Part of your research should include looking at the designer's portfolio. Have they done custom work before? Do you see any items similar to what you're envisioning? Have they previously worked with clients who have your body type? Find and read their custom-order policies as well, if these are publicly available.

- **Get in touch.** Once you've done your research and made a decision, contact the designer. Organize your questions and be succinct and businesslike. Avoid requests for information that can be found easily online. Remember: If a designer's ready to wear pieces are beyond your budget, the custom pieces likely will be as well. And if you know you're not ready to buy, don't waste the designer's time (most custom lingerie designers are small, one-person shops). Questions to ask include how long will it take to construct your item, and what happens if an emergency occurs before the commission is finished and it cannot be completed? Work out all the details in advance, even if it seems awkward. It's better to get the answers you need now rather than later.

- **Have fun with design.** Once you've made your first payment and officially become a client of the designer, it's time to talk the fun stuff—the actual design. Communicate all the ideas from your research to the designer, being as clear and specific as possible. Talk about colors, feelings, moods, where you plan to wear the item, and the types of fabrics you like. The designer may also want more specifics regarding your body type, measurements, or proportions. If the initial design or idea isn't feeling right, let the designer know so you can fix things at this stage. Once the designer begins sewing, any changes will likely incur additional fees.

- **Wait**. After you've both settled and agreed upon the design, then comes the hard part—waiting. You've already discussed a timeline with your designer, so be patient and let the magic happen. You'll be responsible for giving the designer up-to-date measurements, including any changes that may occur while the work is in progress. If things change during this period (for example, you lose or gain weight or you become pregnant), let the designer know as soon as possible so you can discuss any potential alterations.

After you receive your custom creation, enjoy your garment! You're now the proud owner of a truly one-of-kind piece. Remember that it is handmade, and some slight differences between what you saw in the initial sketch and what you receive are normal. And, of course, if you had a great experience, tell your friends! Word of mouth is the most powerful testimonial, especially for small businesses, and your experience can help others take part in the joy of custom lingerie as well.

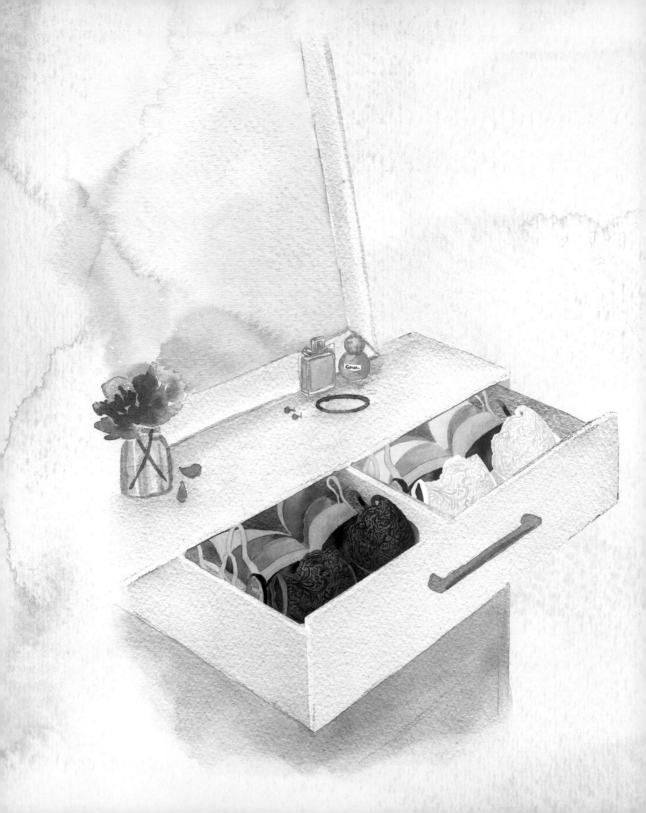

CHAPTER 7

CARE & STORAGE

While knowing how to buy lingerie is important, knowing how to care for and store it is just as essential. It's no good to invest in timeless, well-fitting pieces only to ruin them through improper care and storage.

Knowing how to wash, organize, store, and pack your lingerie will help all your pieces last longer, protecting your investment in yourself. Self-care is something people talk about a lot right now, and caring for your undergarments is a valuable way of caring for yourself.

A Brief History of Lingerie Washing

The history of laundry is in some ways a history of lingerie washing. Because fine fabrics like taffeta, damask, brocade, and velvet couldn't be washed, one's underclothes were critical to keeping outerwear both clean and sweet-smelling.

Lye was one of the first laundry detergents. One of the reasons linen underclothes were especially favored during the Middle Ages is because the fibers could hold up to the harsh stain- and grease-fighting power of dissolved lye (a substance so corrosive it can burn the skin).

However, lye is also the reason so many historical undergarments were white, cream, or other near-white colors. Lye was a powerful bleaching agent, and while it was perfect for making dingy underwear bright again, its effects on dyed underwear were less desirable. By the end of the 1800s, factory-made soaps were everywhere, and these gentler suds could be used on colorful lingerie without fear.

While the very first detergents were developed in the 1930s, World War II stimulated detergent technology, and special intimates washes began to appear in the 1930s and 1940s. By the 1950s, detergents had surpassed laundry soap for wardrobe care, as they allowed people to wash delicate items like nylon, silk, and wool at home without fear of shrinking or fading them.

While you could still use soap or even regular laundry detergent to wash your lingerie, I recommend trying a special intimates wash instead. As I will discuss in more detail, most detergents are too harsh for the fine satin, lace, and elastic of lingerie. Harsh detergents shorten the life expectancy of these fragile fibers. Think of lingerie wash as a gift to yourself that will let you wear your favorite pieces for weeks, months, and years to come.

Why Hand Wash Your Lingerie?

You've probably heard that for lingerie, hand washing is best, and that is completely true. However, I also like to balance that with a dose of reality. Some—not all!—of your pieces will be just fine if you run them through a washing machine. Keep reading to learn what's best for your lingerie wardrobe.

At first glance, the idea of hand washing seems tedious and time-consuming. We're all busy people, and one of the miracles of the modern era is that most of us don't have to spend an entire day hand washing our clothes anymore. That said, washing by hand is honestly better for your undergarments, and the good news is that it doesn't have to be complicated. Let's talk about all the reasons why you should hand wash your lingerie—if you are able to.

First, lingerie is incredibly delicate. While we make many demands on our underwear (comfort, support, and hopefully even a little bit of style), the truth is, lingerie is made from fragile, highly specialized materials that need to be soft enough to wear against the skin but also strong enough to perform a job. Bras are especially difficult items to get right, and a rough tumble in the washer or dryer can twist underwires, pop seams, and permanently distort fabrics.

In fact, I'd say the dryer is even *worse* than the washing machine. Why? Because heat ruins elastic. And once the elastic is ruined, your lingerie is officially dead. Lingerie with ruined elastic won't recover or *snap back*. Instead, your undergarments will stay stretched out, warped, and baggy. Why spend your hard-earned money on exquisite lingerie or high-quality shapewear only to ruin it with a trip through the dryer?

How to Hand Wash Lingerie

I like to break down my hand washing into eight easy steps. That may sound like a lot, but I promise they don't take much work. As an added incentive, you'll be rewarded with gorgeously clean intimates that will maintain their beauty, shape, and elasticity. Here's what to do when lingerie laundry day comes around.

1. Gather your pieces, sorting them by color. Any black, dark, or brightly colored lingerie (like a red bra) will need to be washed separately from your lighter-colored items, because dye can seep out of fabrics and stain the water (which means it might also stain your lingerie).

2. Fill a clean basin, tub, or even a plastic bucket (again, *make sure it's clean*) with lukewarm water. I use a plastic cat-litter pan (don't worry: it's only ever been used to wash lingerie!) because it's cheap, easy to clean, and a good size for holding several pieces at once. The lukewarm water temperature is very important. If anything, err on the side of slightly too cool rather than too hot. Note: If you're washing blood out of underwear, use ice-cold water. Hot or warm water will set stains into the fibers, and you won't be able to remove them. You may also want to use hydrogen peroxide or a hydrogen peroxide–based cleanser, such as OxiClean, in place of step 3.

3. Add your detergent to the basin. As I mentioned earlier, I recommend a special lingerie or delicates wash. If that's not an option, use a gentle laundering agent like Marseille soap, castile soap, or baby shampoo. The point is to not use harsh detergents or soaps, which have added chemicals and could possibly ruin your fabrics. Avoid washing-machine detergents or bleach-containing products as well. When adding your lingerie wash to the sink, a little goes a long way. One teaspoon per gallon is a good guideline. Too much lingerie wash and you may have trouble rinsing it all out at the end.

4. Once you've added your lingerie wash, submerge your pieces in the soapy water. Agitate the water a little with your hands—nothing too dramatic, just a light stirring motion (I drag my hand through the water in the shape of a figure 8). You may also want to lightly squeeze your lingerie to ensure the sudsy water

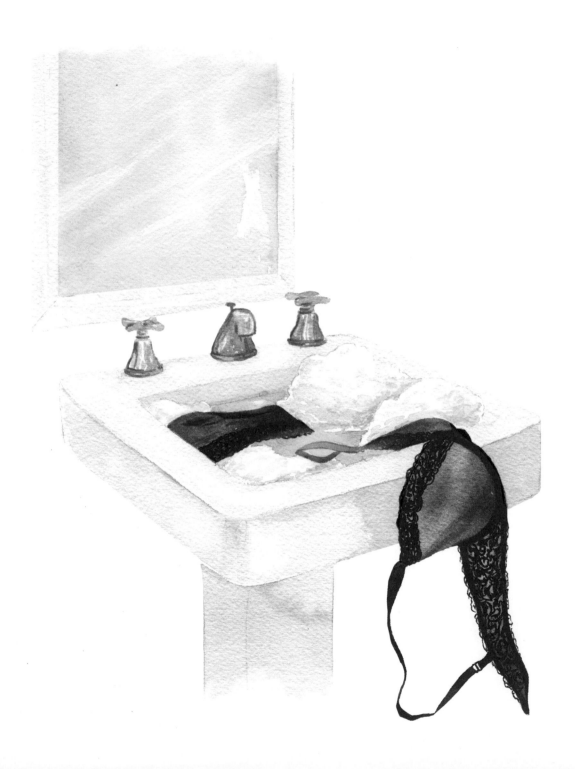

gets incorporated into the fibers. Then leave everything to soak for fifteen minutes or so (longer if heavily soiled).

5. After the allotted time, hand clean any areas needing extra attention. I find a soft-bristled toothbrush is good for underwear gussets and other areas that may need a light scrubbing.

6. Rinse your lingerie until you're sure it's free of cleanser. Some people like to drain the sink or empty the tub and refill it with fresh water for this step. Unless you're using a no-rinse wash, make sure the water rinses clear and suds-free before moving on.

7. Lightly squeeze any excess water out of your lingerie. Don't wring, don't twist, and don't ball it up. Be gentle here. You don't want to risk bending a wire or popping a seam.

8. Now you can hang your lingerie to air dry or lightly press it between two clean, dry towels. You can also lay your garments flat on a clean towel instead of hanging them up (hanging may cause some items to stretch out). However, make sure you reshape padded or contour cup bras before setting them out to dry so no permanent dents take hold in the fabric. And make sure your lingerie isn't hanging over a heater!

That's it! You're done! The most important steps are leaving your lingerie to soak, rinsing it well, and then drying it appropriately. I wash my lingerie about once per week. To me, it's meditative, and I'll also put on a face mask and brew a cup of tea during the process. You might want to take a walk or watch your favorite show while your underthings are getting clean. It's so easy and adds to the life of your garments.

HOW OFTEN SHOULD YOU WASH YOUR LINGERIE?

TYPE OF LINGERIE	WASH FREQUENCY
Knickers	After each wear
Bras	Every two to three wears. You'll want to wash them more often if they're dirty or sweaty or if you have sensitive skin or a skin condition. Note: Washing too often can damage the bra's elasticity, ruining it prematurely.
Sports bras	After each wear
Hosiery	After each wear
Pajamas, nightwear, loungewear	Once per week (roughly every four to five wears)

How to Machine Wash Lingerie

While hand washing is best, sometimes life gets in the way and you simply don't have the time. But your intimates still need to get clean. Keep in mind that some items, like cotton panties and undershirts, are just fine after a trip through the washing machine. Other items, like a lace chemise or silk camisole, could be permanently destroyed. While I am all about being practical and real when it comes to lingerie washing, you also want to use your common sense. If something is light, flimsy, or delicate to the touch, it might not survive even one trip in the washing machine. With that in mind, here are a few things to know when machine washing so you don't completely wreck your undergarments.

1. As with hand washing, sort items into dark and light colors.
2. Use a lingerie wash bag. Use *several* lingerie wash bags if you need to.

3. As with hand washing, use a specialty lingerie wash or gentle soap instead of a conventional laundry detergent.

4. If using a washing machine for your intimates, your lingerie should be the only items in there. *Don't* wash your lingerie with your other clothes and especially not with heavy garments like blankets, towels, or jeans. That may mean your washing machine is only a quarter full. That's fine. Having more empty space reduces the likelihood of damaged undergarments.

5. Choose the cold water and delicate cycles on the machine.

6. Once the wash cycle is over, hang more delicate items to dry. Cotton and microfiber underwear is usually fine in the dryer so long as it's on a low or cool setting (they won't last as long as they would if air dried, but underwear tends to be more replaceable than bras). Never put items with high spandex or elastic content (shapewear, stretch lace thongs, etc.) in the dryer. Bras also should never be machine dried. Finally, don't machine dry any kind of hosiery and never tumble dry silk or embroidered, embellished, or appliquéd items.

Dry Cleaning Lingerie

I know, I know . . . you're probably rolling your eyes but hear me out: some items should *only* be dry cleaned. If an item says "dry clean only," you should probably follow that advice. Some experts think you can take a chance with hand washing, but honestly, why risk ruining that expensive, once-in-a-lifetime purchase? Dry cleaning is pricey, but having to throw something away because you destroyed it costs even more.

You're most likely to need a dry cleaner for items like silk robes or gowns and steel-boned corsets (which should *never* be submerged in water). Long, delicate lace pieces may also be better left to the dry cleaners. Silk bras and knickers can be gently hand washed, but you'll want to keep an eye on them. Soaking too long can make the silk lose its luster, or, even worse, cause the dye to bleed if there's a print. Similar to vintage lingerie, I'd even recommend doing a spot test first, just to be sure the water won't damage the fabric.

BONUS TIP

Looking to save some drying time? A salad spinner can gently draw the excess water out of your bras, helping them dry faster!

When choosing a dry cleaning service for your lingerie, make sure they have experience in cleaning your specific type of item. This isn't the time to experiment with a random dry cleaner just because they dropped a coupon in your mailbox. If an item is especially delicate or embellished, ask if the cleaner has experience with bridal gowns or evening wear; a similarly gentle touch is necessary for those kinds of elaborate garments.

As a brief aside, to spot clean a corset, spray a 1:1 mixture of vodka and water on the *interior*. Leave it out for a night, and it will dry without an odor.

Now that all your lingerie is clean and fresh, it's time to get it organized!

How to Organize & Store Lingerie

I don't know about you, but organizing my lingerie is one of the hardest things to do. I like how easy it is to see everything once it's all in its place (being able to pull out my favorite bra in an instant is a definite plus), but getting there can be daunting.

Bras, panties, slips . . . they're all small things, and that can make them harder to keep track of. Worse yet, poorly storing your lingerie can lead to issues like permanently dented cups, wrinkled and creased lingerie, or, in the very worst cases, moth-eaten or moldy undergarments. It makes me feel depressed just thinking about it! In this section, you'll learn how to store your everyday things and get some tips and tricks for taking care of your more special-occasion garments.

The first step in organizing your lingerie is to get rid of *everything* you don't wear. I was going to say "everything you don't love," but realistically speaking, I don't *love* my T-shirt bras, yet I wear them all the time, so let's be practical here. When I say get rid of everything you don't wear, I mean *be absolutely ruthless*. If it hasn't seen the light of day in a year, it doesn't belong in your underwear drawer. If it's scratchy, itchy, or uncomfortable, toss it. If it feels weird when you put it on, it has to go. If it's in a size that you aspire to be, not the one you actually are, stop torturing yourself and get rid of it. It's so much better to have a lingerie drawer full (or even half full) of things you're excited about wearing and that fit you, as opposed to drawer full of "maybe someday" garments.

I also suggest getting rid of anything old, misshapen, discolored, ratty, torn, or that has otherwise seen better days. The one possible exception is underwear you only wear during your period, but truthfully, I think it's better to just invest in seven pairs of plain black knickers, if you can. Wearing discolored, stretched out, uncomfortable underwear doesn't make anyone feel good. It also means your lingerie probably isn't doing its job.

Take a bra, for example. As we discussed back in chapter 1, most of the support comes from the band. That means, once the band is stretched out, that bra is no longer doing its job of supporting your bust. When that happens, it's time to trash the bra. Also say your good-byes to anything with holes in it or missing underwires. Set your standards high. You deserve to wear beautiful, comfortable, and supportive lingerie, not underwear that's seen better days and makes you feel terrible.

If you have anything brand new—and I mean *brand new, never worn*—with the tags still attached, consider donating it. Lingerie is expensive, and that set you never got around to wearing could be exactly what someone else needs. However, please don't donate anything that's been worn. You wouldn't want to wear dirty, used underwear, and neither does anyone else.

Next, group your lingerie into categories. There are a few different ways to do this. One possible method is to sort everything into everyday, sport, and special-occasion categories. Another grouping strategy is to sort by colors, such as black, skin tone, brights, and prints. You could also try sorting by bra sets, loungewear, and sexy pieces. There's any number of ways to tackle this part. You'll know what's best for you. In my case, I have a drawer for everyday lingerie, a drawer for hosiery, a drawer for special-occasion items, and a drawer for swimwear and athletic wear. I also hang my fanciest robes in the closet. Whatever method you use, you want to be able to easily find what you wear most often, but you also want your nice pieces to be visible and not get lost, especially as you get more confidence in wearing lingerie.

At this point, a lot of people would recommend drawer dividers or underwear organizers. Those are both great options if you like them, but I prefer to just fold my underwear and put it directly in the drawer (I also like to place a little lavender sachet or a few dryer sheets in my lingerie drawer to impart a light, pleasant scent to my underthings). With my bras, I simply lay them flat with the cups stacked atop each other. Some people fold their bras to save space, but if you fold a contour cup or padded bra, you may find the foam gets dented (see the bonus tip on page 38 for advice on removing dents from foam cups). Nonpadded bras or bralettes are fine to fold, however.

You also want to fasten your bra hooks before putting your bras away. Hooks can snag on delicate materials, tearing the lingerie you've taken such good care of. One thing to remember: make sure the inside of your underwear drawer is smooth to the touch. If there's any roughness at all, it either needs to be addressed or the drawers should be lined with something smooth, like contact paper or wallpaper.

For long, delicate items, such as gowns made from silk chiffon or items too bulky for drawers, such as flannel or fleece pajamas, hang them in your closet. The exception to this is heavily embellished lingerie (for example, a bed jacket decorated with feathers and sequins) or bias-cut lingerie. Heavy items can tear themselves apart when hung and bias-cut items can warp as gravity works on the seams. For pieces like these, carefully fold them, place them between sheets of acid-free tissue paper, and keep them in a drawer that's exclusively for your most delicate pieces (this is also a good idea for your vintage lingerie). Use good-quality, padded hangers and perhaps even place your nicer pieces in a garment bag with a few cedar balls to ensure they're in good shape when you're ready to wear them again.

And that's it! You're done organizing!

Now that you've gotten rid of all the stuff you don't like and have a better sense of what you wear all the time, use that knowledge to inform your next lingerie purchases. You are worth a lingerie wardrobe full of nothing but the good stuff. And by good stuff, I don't mean the most expensive stuff, but the stuff that meets your

BONUS TIP

Always wash your lingerie before wearing it for the first time. Not only do you not know who may have tried it on before, but you also want to wash off any factory residues left over from the manufacturing process.

needs and makes you feel amazing and glorious and confident. It doesn't matter if it's popular or trendy or if it's the same bra you already own five of. If it makes you feel good and you wear it all the time, get more of it. You'll thank yourself later.

How to Pack Lingerie for Travel

We've all heard horror stories of suitcases being mangled on the runway or disappearing all together on the way to your destination. The most important things when packing lingerie for travel (whether the trip is for business or pleasure) are to make sure your lingerie arrives where you are and intact. The next most important thing is to make sure you don't overpack. Those luggage fees can be brutal, and wouldn't you rather have that money for souvenirs? Here's how I approach packing my lingerie when it's time for a trip.

- **Plan your lingerie like you plan your outfits**. You won't be able to bring everything, so be deliberate and make sure you bring underthings appropriate for your activities at the destination. Going backpacking for a couple of weeks? Moisture-wicking sports bras and knickers, which can be washed in a sink and hung to dry, might be best. Spending seventeen hours on a flight halfway around the world? Don't subject yourself to shapewear or a brand-new and untested bra. Instead, maybe bring a pair of lounge pants and an eye mask to relax in later! Honeymoon time? Well, first, congratulations! Second, don't forget your most showstopping pieces. This is the perfect occasion for them!

- **Always pack an emergency lingerie set in your carry-on bag**. I suggest choosing a fresh pair of underwear, a clean bra, and a pair of socks. This is your layover insurance. I travel often, and I've had to deal with canceled flights, weather delays, and one-hour layovers that turned into twelve-hour ones. When you're stressed and frustrated, even a small thing like a clean pair of socks can make your day a little brighter. And, real talk: Accidents happen. Your period might start early. Someone might spill a drink on you. You might get sick. Whatever the situation, at least you'll be covered.

- **Bring enough underwear.** A good rule of thumb is to bring as many knickers as there are days you'll be traveling (up to seven pairs total). For example, when I backpacked across Europe in my twenties, I purchased a week's worth of high-quality, sweat-wicking knickers, handwashed them in the evenings, and they lasted me my entire trip. For bras, I recommend the number of days of your trip divided by two (up to five bras total). That way, you'll never have to wear the same bra twice in a row and you'll have enough bras to be able to wash a few at a time and avoid running out. Finally, pack a little lingerie wash with you as well. Even if it's a short trip, you never know when you might need it. No matter what, never pack just one bra and one pair of panties. Even if you'll only be gone overnight, two is the bare minimum.

- **Pack it right.** When it comes to the actual packing, it's fine to fold or roll your underwear, unpadded bras, and loungewear. Never fold or roll padded or contour cup bras, however. Instead, stack your contour cups. Some people stack vertically, layering their bras directly on top of each other. Others prefer to stack horizontally (so that when you look down, there's a neat row of bras). You might even place your rolled-up socks and knickers in the bra cups so the cups don't become crushed. Just don't undo your work by placing something heavy, like shoes or jeans, on top of them.

- **Unpack with care.** Once you get to your destination, don't forget to hang up certain items (like that beautiful robe or gown). Also, do a quick wardrobe check to make sure all your lingerie arrived safe and sound.

Conclusion

When I first became interested in lingerie, I didn't understand its power or appeal. All my life, I'd assumed lingerie was something to wear for other people—for a romantic partner to appreciate or to help ensure I looked professional for a job interview. But no one ever told me that lingerie could be for myself, that it could be a way to explore my identity, my personality, my sense of style, and my interests.

In our day-to-day lives, we're told that the purpose of lingerie is to help us look slimmer or younger, to give us the "right" shape under our clothes, or to hide what the rest of society perceives as blemishes or flaws. And lingerie can do all that. But it's limiting and unsatisfying to think of lingerie solely in terms of ways it can help us "fix" our bodies. There's nothing exciting, nothing inspiring, about wearing lingerie just so your body can look "okay."

I believe lingerie, at its heart, should be a way for us to explore ourselves—our possibilities, potential, and personhood. I know I must sound strange right now, but think about it. We all have outfits or uniforms we have to wear for the outside world. Sometimes, as in the case of the military or first responders, that's a literal uniform. But more often, it's symbolic: we're told that we're *supposed* to dress a certain way, and so we do it, whether we feel personally inspired or motivated to dress in that manner or not.

But lingerie, our intimate apparel, the clothing we wear against our skin that no one else has to see, well, that can be our truest expression of self. Our lingerie can be a place to play, to experiment, to examine what you love and discover what you hate. Dreaming of a trip to Paris? Wear French lingerie. Love the pinup look? Adopt it with a garter belt. Want to feel like a movie star? Indulge in a floor-length satin robe. Chasing a toddler? Get in touch with yourself again through soft, romantic lace.

The possibilities of lingerie are truly endless. But you have to know what you're looking for and the language to use to find what you want. You have to know the difference between a bustier and a demi cup so that you can describe the lingerie you want to buy, and the difference between silk and satin so that when you're ready to splurge, you're buying exactly what you desire. You have to know how to take care of your new and special and extraordinary purchases so you don't lose heart before you've barely begun. And you've got to give yourself time. Allow yourself—*gift* yourself—permission to be curious, to delight in satin and lace, and to feel joy about a beautiful print or an impeccably stitched seam.

So often, we're encouraged to put ourselves last. To put our needs, wants, and desires after everyone else's. But lingerie is a way of putting yourself first. It's a way of taking care of yourself, treating yourself, and nourishing yourself. You deserve to celebrate your body and delight in your lingerie, to pamper and spoil yourself with the very best underwear you can afford. Don't let anyone tell you different or convince you that you're not worth it. You deserve the most beautiful lingerie in the world, and I hope this book helps you discover that.

Lingerie is a world full of possibilities. Enjoy it.

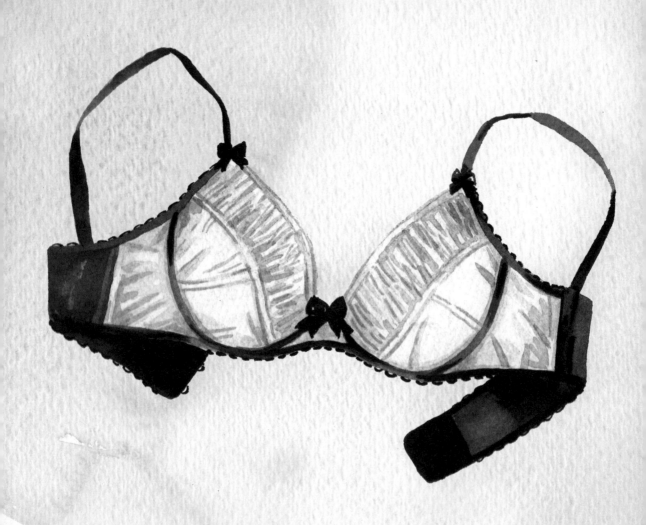

Special Bra-Fitting Concerns

Chapter 1 covered the basics of bra fitting, but if you have a special fit or body concern, this appendix is for you.

Plus Size

You may find that you need to size down from your underbust measurements for an ideal fit. There are two reasons for this. One, you may have more "squish" around your rib cage. This means that your band will need to be a little tighter to anchor properly and also that you may be able to tolerate a tighter band (and therefore a more secure fit) than someone whose bra band rests directly on the bones of the rib cage. Two, bra bands, especially in modern-day bras, are stretchy. The longer the band (that is, the larger the band size), the more stretchy the band is. This is due to a quirk of elastic fabrics; essentially, more stretch fabric equals more stretch. If you are plus-sized and small busted, you likely wear a hard-to-find size. Sister sizing down one band size and up one cup size (and then using a bra band extender, if applicable) may offer a wider range of fashionable options.

Trans Women & Nonbinary People

If you are transitioning or getting ready to buy your first bra, it can be a daunting step. While you might be just fine going braless for a while, many transitioning people find they need bras once their nipples become more visible and projected or once they have enough breast tissue to bounce while running or going up and down stairs. Even if you're not developing breasts at the moment or have no interest in hormone replacement therapy (HRT) or mammoplasty, bras can help with gender dysphoria.

As with all bra-fitting methods, you'll need to know your measurements. While some experts recommend going with your exact rib-cage measure for the bra band, if you're transitioning from an Assigned Male at Birth body (AMAB), you'll almost certainly want to size up by two or even four inches (or potentially more, depending on your body shape and comfort level). This is especially true at first, as bras can take time to get used to. If you have a wider rib cage, perhaps with more muscle and less "squish," a larger size can help you avoid any discomfort from the bra band digging into your ribs. If you don't yet have a lot of breast tissue to support, the band is also doing less "work," which means it doesn't need to fit as snugly.

Contour cup plunge bras and bras with push-up style padding can help shape and project the bust and also makes it easier to add optional bra pads or inserts (also known as *cookies*). However, if that's not comfortable for you (or if you'd rather wear a bra without padding), bralettes are a good choice. Because bralettes tend to come in small, medium, and large sizes instead of cup and band sizes, and because they have unstructured cups, bralettes can be more size-flexible as well as more accommodating to a developing bust.

Last, if you have just started HRT, avoid running out and buying a lot of bras right away. Your bra size will likely change often in the next few weeks to months, and you may experience some pain and sensitivity as well. If that's the case, look for bras with soft interior linings to avoid irritation.

Mastectomy/Post-Surgery

A mastectomy bra is designed specifically for people who have undergone mastectomies (the surgical removal of one or both breasts). While many mastectomy bras have pockets to accommodate a breast form, an increasing number of mastectomy bras are pocketless or made with only minimal or light padding for people who prefer to go "unpocketed." Mastectomy bras are also wireless and tend to be made with wider, more stabilizing sides to keep the bra in place and help center the remaining breast tissue or breast form.

Before purchasing a mastectomy bra, it can be especially useful to go to a professional bra fitter or seek the guidance of a mastectomy expert. You'll also want to give yourself enough time after surgery for your chest to heal before beginning the search for a mastectomy bra.

Some things to keep in mind, especially if your surgery is recent: Breast forms and breast reconstructions don't behave the same as natural breasts. The softness you may have been used to from your own breast tissue won't be present in a breast form or breast reconstruction. You may also find that you need to go up a band size, either to avoid irritating your scar tissue or to accommodate the extra mass of breast forms. More than anything, make sure your bra is comfortable, which might mean wearing a soft, lightly structured bralette or even a post-surgical bra. You don't want to put yourself at risk for infection, irritation, or swelling due to an errant seam or clasp.

Maternity & Nursing

Gone are the days of boring, ugly maternity bras. Now many bra brands have expanded into maternity styles, offering fun, fashionable options for expectant and nursing parents.

Maternity bras tend to have stretchy, size-flexible cups as well as softly lined interiors. They also tend to have more hook-and-eye closures at the back to accommodate an expanding rib cage and straps with greater adjustability. While maternity bras are made for wearing during your pregnancy, nursing bras are made for those who are breast-feeding. The key feature of a nursing bra is a latch or clasp on each cup that allows the baby to access the breast and nipple for feeding.

You can expect to buy several bras over the course of your pregnancy. Your breasts will increase in size and weight (usually by a couple of pounds or so), and that means you will likely go up a few cup sizes. You will want to purchase your first maternity bra around week 10, close to the end of the first trimester. This is the end of a period of major breast growth, and you'll almost certainly have sized out of all your other bras. Around week 20, you'll want to do another bra buy. Finally, in the third trimester, around week 30, you'll want to transition from maternity bras to nursing bras if you haven't already done so.

Some people say not to wear an underwire when nursing, however, underwires in and of themselves are not dangerous to a lactating breast. The issue is that many people either don't have access to the size they need or don't purchase the size they need. In those cases, the wire can sit atop the breast tissue, which is not only uncomfortable, but can also lead to painful complications such as mastitis. Also, buy the best quality you can afford. Your maternity bras will undergo a lot of use and need a lot of washing. Both you and the baby will appreciate it.

You'll want to have a minimum of three nursing bras to start. One you can wash, one you can wear, and one on standby. Keep in mind that at six weeks after birth, twelve weeks after birth, and six months after birth, your breasts may be looking and feeling very different, so don't buy too many bras at the very beginning.

When measuring for your new nursing bra size, measure at engorgement (when your breasts are at their fullest). That's the size you want to buy so that there's enough cup volume to accommodate the breast as it fills and there are no pressure points.

One final thing: Your breasts won't be the same after pregnancy and nursing. You can keep wearing your maternity bras for a while after you've stopped nursing, and they may be useful as your breasts gradually shrink in size during weaning. Some people even keep their maternity bras as sleep or lounge bras.

Fibromyalgia & Skin Sensitivity

Wearing a bra when you feel achy all over or when your skin is sensitive can be torture. While going braless or wearing a camisole are certainly options (see "Braless Options" on page 20 for more suggestions), it's not for everyone. Soft, breathable natural fabrics are your friends. Avoid artificial fibers that may irritate your skin or exacerbate an attack. Look for fabrics made from rayon (also known as modal, tencel, bamboo, or viscose), silk, cotton, and linen (see page 50 for more about the specific qualities of these fibers). Keep an eye out for bras that bill themselves as hypoallergenic and then do the touch test, if you can, to get a sense of the bra's *hand* (see page 98 for more on "hand"). If the material feels rough to your fingers, it will feel even worse on your body. Simple, minimalist underpinnings, such as those without lace trim, are also a good idea. Seams and underwires may be a source of irritation, which means wirefree bralettes with soft cups are an excellent option to try. If you find you absolutely must wear an underwire bra, look for ones with soft interior linings and padded underwires to lessen pain, irritation, and flare-ups. Also, check the center gore to make sure it's covered in soft fabric.

Loungewear items such as slips and camisoles are another possible bra alternative, especially if these items have shaped cups. If you struggle with fibromyalgia and have difficulty with mobility and dexterity (such as with reaching behind your back), also keep an eye out for front-closure bras, as they may be easier to manage.

Finally, when you wash your bras, use a sensitive-skin detergent or specialty lingerie wash without additives or enzymes. *Plain*, *gentle*, and *unscented* are all good words to know. You may also find that washing your bras after every wear helps cut down on flare-ups and skin irritation.

Augmented Breasts

The first thing to remember is that breasts with implants don't "behave" the same way as breasts without them. Right after surgery, don't worry about buying new bras. Instead, give your breasts and chest time to heal with post-surgery bras and then soft, underwire-free bras. Wait until the swelling is completely gone and your implants "settle" before bra shopping.

The next thing to remember is that breast implants are not sized according to cup sizes. They reference cubic centimeters, which is a volume measurement. It's important to measure yourself after surgery because what looks like a C cup to your eyes might actually be a D, E, or F cup once you perform the measurement techniques described on page 17.

Your breasts may also be a different shape post-augmentation, such as full all around instead of full on bottom or pendulous. This new shape will affect which bras are now most comfortable for you. However, your band size, since it's based on your rib cage measurement, will most likely be the same or close to the same as before the augmentation.

Keep in mind that your breast size and shape will continue changing throughout the first year or two, so don't buy too many bras to start. Give your body time to get used to the implants (this is sometimes referred to as "dropping"), and don't be surprised if the bras you buy right after surgery are less comfortable six months down the road. That's perfectly normal.

Physical Disabilities

A few paragraphs can't possibly do justice to this topic, since there are dozens, if not hundreds, of potential mobility and fit concerns that apply to persons with disabilities. However, here are a few more general tips centered specifically around physical accessibility and daily bra wear.

- **Front-closure bras:** These tend to work especially well for those with limited mobility or joint stiffness (as with arthritis). In addition to the usual front hook-and-eye styles, also look for bras with Velcro, snap, or even magnetic closures, all of which are easier to manage if you have limited use of your hands.

- **Bras without fasteners:** Bras such as those you can slip over your head or step into and work up your body are another option. For this style especially, look for stretch jersey or knit fabrics such as microfiber, as they'll not only be easier to pull on, but will also retain their shape better. Depending on the level of support you prefer, pullover-style bralettes or even adhesive bras are a potential option as well.

- **Bra tools:** Consider using a tool like the Bra Angel, which is meant to allow for one-handed bra fastening (particularly useful for amputees or people who can use only one hand). The Bra Angel works by holding one end of the bra securely in place while you bring the other end around to fasten.

- **Customization:** Some independent designers or small brands may also be able to customize a bra specifically for your needs (see page 103 for more info on custom-lingerie shopping).

Binders

Binding is a transformative experience that can help you cope with dysphoria and give your body the shape you desire, but it's important to bind safely. Using elastic bandages or tape to bind is incredibly dangerous and can be hazardous to your health, causing scarring, lung problems, and even broken ribs. A store-bought binder, while more expensive, can be easier to use and is also safer.

The first thing you'll need to know for your binder is your measurements. Measure across the fullest or widest part of your chest (this is usually right under your armpits, about nipple height). The tape should be snug, but it shouldn't compress or dig into the tissue. Be upright; don't slouch over or project your chest outward. It's very important this measurement be accurate. If you can, get a friend to help.

Binders are made to flatten or compress the chest, so even if it sounds like a good idea to go down one size from what the brand's sizing chart recommends, don't. You should be able to breathe while wearing a binder. If it makes you feel lightheaded or hurts, take it off! If you're on the borderline between sizes or unsure about sizing, it doesn't hurt to email the company and get their advice.

You shouldn't wear a binder more than eight to twelve hours a day. Don't wear your binder overnight or during heavy physical activity, such as exercise.

Binders tend to come in two lengths: half (ending around the middle of the rib cage) and full (covering the stomach). If binders aren't available to you, know that some people compress their chest with sports bras. Look for sports bras that give a smooth look across the chest.

Finally, don't forget to wash your binder regularly. Because of their elastic nature, binders don't do well in the washer and dryer. Hand wash with a mild detergent and warm water and then hang to dry.

Special Underwear Concerns

While chapter 2 covers the basics of underwear, those with more specific concerns may find this section useful.

Menstruation

Many lingerie brands now offer underwear specifically to wear during your period. These knickers are made with absorbent gussets meant to be used alone on lighter flow days or as a backup to a primary method of menstrual care, such as a pad, tampon, or menstrual cup. Many styles suitable for menstruation are also absorbent enough to help with light incontinence, a common issue after childbirth and menopause.

Pregnancy

During your prenatal period, you may find underwear that goes under the baby bump to be more comfortable than styles with a higher waistband (unless the waistband goes all the way over your bump). Look for lower-rise underwear like hipsters and bikinis. You may find you need to go up a size or two from your nonpregnancy size, especially later in the term. If you find you need more support for the belly, maternity underwear with a stretch panel over the abdomen can be useful. You can also look into side-tie or side-closure underwear, especially for later in the pregnancy when you may have trouble bending over. It's more important than ever not to buy underwear that's too tight, as this can affect circulation, which can potentially injure you or your baby! After pregnancy, many people continue to wear their maternity underwear or other high-waisted styles.

Menopause

Hot flashes and night sweats tend to be a major issue for people undergoing menopause, which makes underwear with moisture-wicking technology especially useful. The skin of the vulva can also become thin, delicate, or sensitive during menopause. Choosing underwear made from soft, skin-friendly materials and breathable natural fibers like cotton and silk can help. In addition, not wearing underwear at night is an option.

Vulvodynia

Characterized by persistent, unexplained pain in the vulva, vulvodynia can feel like a constant, burning sensation or can only flare-up when there's pressure on the genitals (such as through tampon use or sexual activity). If you struggle with this condition, look for loose-fitting underwear made from natural fibers. Tap shorts, boyshorts, and even long pantalettes and bloomers are all options, so long as they're made from fibers like cotton, silk, or bamboo. Avoid thongs or underwear made from synthetic materials, such as nylon or polyester. Switching to detergents specially made for sensitive skin can help avoid irritation. Finally, when shopping for underwear, pay special attention to seams, specifically those on or near the gusset.

Trans Women & Nonbinary People

Our underwear is an expression of our identity, and your underwear should reflect who you are. If you have external genitalia and prefer more feminine styles, avoid buying cheap, tight underwear made from synthetic materials. Though it may seem good for keeping everything contained, synthetics don't allow air to flow well and that, combined with tightness, could lead to issues with circulation and infection. Boyshorts and boxers made from breathable fabrics with a bit of stretch are good at giving room for your body while helping blur your silhouette, if that's something you want. High-waisted briefs and hip-hugger styles with wider sides are also good for this, especially if you prefer tucking. If you're between sizes, consider sizing up to take into account the differences in proportions. Shapewear and panties with a built-in gaff are also potential solutions. However, avoid doubling up on underwear, wearing underwear that's too small, or using tape. Some indie designers are able to customize underwear to help you during your transition.

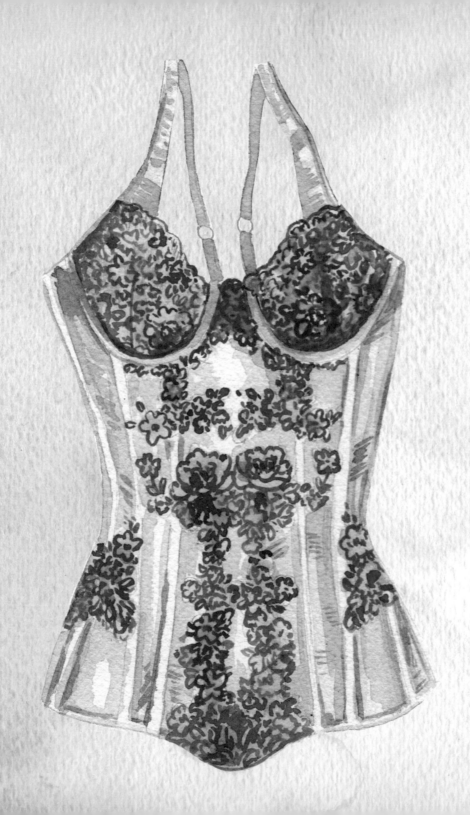

Sample Lingerie Wardrobes

You know the basics of lingerie and you're ready to shop, but maybe you need a little nudge to know where to start or how to put together the lingerie wardrobe of your dreams. Take a look at these sample wardrobes (ranging from your basic, everyday lingerie collection to an extravagant, luxury lingerie wardrobe!) for suggestions.

Fifteen-Piece Lingerie Basics Wardrobe

- **Bras (four):** One assortment could include a T-shirt bra, a bralette, a convertible bra, and a strapless bra. Or you could replace two of those with a bustier for special occasions and a sports bra.

- **Knickers (six):** One per day until the weekend. For extra versatility, choose seamless styles to go under the widest range of clothing.

- **Shapewear (one):** In addition to shaping and smoothing, shapewear can be worn as an extra thermal layer. Opt for a shaping slip or high-waisted shaping shorts for maximum flexibility.

- **Hosiery (two):** One pair of nude pantyhose in your skin tone and one pair of opaque black tights is a good place to start.

- **Loungewear/sleepwear (two):** One chemise or pajama set to wear to bed, and one robe for wearing around the house is a good duo. You can also replace one of these items with a camisole for more versatility.

Twelve-Piece Honeymoon/Bridal Wardrobe

- **Matching sets (three sets, six items total):** These are splurgeworthy and luxurious.

- **Nightgowns or chemise (two):** Essentially, you want something comfortable to wear around your honeymoon suite, so pack a nightgown and a chemise. Or you can substitute, selecting one or two from a romper, lounge set, camisole and shorts set, or pajama set . . . preferably in silk!

- **Robe (one):** You'll be spending a lot of time in your room, so a robe you'll enjoy slipping into is nice to have on hand. As an added bonus, you'll remember your honeymoon whenever you wear it again.

- **Boudoir slippers (one pair):** Your honeymoon is the perfect time for a pair of marabou feather pumps, silk lounge slippers, or whatever else your heart desires.

- **Showstopping ensembles (two):** Wow your partner. Then wow your partner again. Think drama—the bigger, the better.

Thirty-Piece Luxury Lingerie Wardrobe

- **Bras (five):** One possible combination is two everyday T-shirt bras, two sports bras, and one convertible/strapless bra. (You can also substitute one of these with a bralette or lounge bra if you also want a less structured option.)

- **Knickers (five):** Everyday styles that work under a wide range of clothing are best.

- **Matching sets (three sets, six items total):** Treat yourself to the ultimate lingerie indulgence—three matching bra and panty sets. Nothing makes you feel more put together and in charge of your life than coordinating underwear.

- **Shapewear (three):** A good assortment for a wide range of wardrobe options could consist of a shaping slip, shaping shorts, and a shaping bodysuit or teddy.

- **Hosiery (five):** A good range for your lingerie wardrobe might be three pairs of everyday basics (such as one pair of skin tone pantyhose, one pair of sheer black pantyhose, and one pair of opaque black tights), plus two pairs of fashion hosiery (such as fishnets, lace tights, or thigh-high stockings).

- **Loungewear/sleepwear (five):** With so much to choose from, you can opt for a seasonal loungewear collection (winter and summer) and even treat yourself to an opulent, deluxe loungewear purchase. I recommend one lightweight knit robe for travel and summer (the thinner fabric makes it easier to pack), one heavy fleece or flannel winter robe, one chemise or nightgown, one pajama set, and one special purchase—whether it's a babydoll, dressing gown, or bed jacket.

- **Wildcard (one):** What's the one thing you've always wanted—a corset, bodysuit, pair of boudoir slippers, vintage slip, retro-inspired girdle, or lingerie dress that can double as outerwear? Use this space to fulfill your wildest lingerie dream.

Bra Size Conversion Charts

INTERNATIONAL BRA CUP SIZE CONVERSION CHART

U.S.	U.K.	E.U.
AA	AA	AA
A	A	A
B	B	B
C	C	C
D	D	D
DD/E	DD	E
DDD/F	E	F
DDDD/G	F	G
DDDDD/H	FF	H
I	G	I
J	GG	J
K	H	K
L	HH	L
M	J	M
N	JJ	N
	K	
	KK	
	L	
	LL	

28	30	32	34	36	38
28A	30AA				
28B	30A	32AA			
28C	30B	32A	34AA		
28D	30C	32B	34A	36AA	
28DD/E	30D	32C	34B	36A	38AA
28DDD/F	30DD/E	32D	34C	36B	38A
28DDDD/G	30DDD/F	32DD/E	34D	36C	38B
28DDDDD/H	30DDDD/G	32DDD/F	34DD/E	36D	38C
28I	30DDDDD/H	32DDDD/G	34DDD/F	36DD/E	38D
28J	30I	32DDDDD/H	34DDDD/G	36DDD/F	38DD/E
28K	30J	32I	34DDDDD/H	36DDDD/G	38DDD/F
28L	30K	32J	34I	36DDDDD/H	38DDDD/G
28M	30L	32K	34J	36I	38DDDDD/H
28N	30M	32L	34K	36J	38I
	30N	32M	34L	36K	38J
		32N	34M	36L	38K
			34N	36M	38L
				36N	38M
					38N

All bra sizes in each row are sister sizes, that is, they are the same cup volume (see page 18). Note: This bra chart uses U.S. bra sizing. To convert these cup sizes to U.K. or E.U. sizing, consult the size chart on page 137.

40	42	44	46	48	50	52
40AA						
40A	42AA					
40B	42A	44AA				
40C	42B	44A	46AA			
40D	42C	44B	46A	48AA		
40DD/E	42D	44C	46B	48A	50AA	
40DDD/F	42DD/E	44D	46C	48B	50A	52AA
40DDDD/G	42DDD/F	44DD/E	46D	48C	50B	52A
40DDDDD/H	42DDDD/G	44DDD/F	46DD/E	48D	50C	52B
40I	42DDDDD/H	44DDDD/G	46DDD/F	48DD/E	50D	52C
40J	42I	44DDDDD/H	46DDDD/G	48DDD/F	50DD/E	52D
40K	42J	44I	46DDDDD/H	48DDDD/G	50DDD/F	52DD/E
40L	42K	44J	46I	48DDDDD/H	50DDDD/G	52DDD/F
40M	42L	44K	46J	48I	50DDDDD/H	52DDDD/G
40N	42M	44L	46K	48J	50I	52DDDDD/H
	42N	44M	46L	48K	50J	52I
		44N	46M	48L	50K	52J
			46N	48M	50L	52K
				48N	50M	52L
					50N	52M
						52N

Further Reading

Bruna, D., and Bard Graduate Center for Studies in the Decorative Arts, eds. 2015. *Fashioning the Body: An Intimate History of the Silhouette*. New Haven, London: Yale University Press.

Chenoune, F. 2005. *Hidden Underneath: A History of Lingerie*. New York: Assouline Publishing.

Cunnington, C. W., and P. Cunnington. 1992. *The History of Underclothes*. Mineola, New York: Dover Publications.

Ewing, E. 1971. *Fashion in Underwear: From Babylon to Bikini Brief*. Mineola, New York: Dover Publications.

Farrell-Beck, J., and C. Gau. 2002. *Uplift: The Bra in America*. Philadelphia: University of Pennsylvania Press.

Field, J. 2007. *An Intimate Affair: Women, Lingerie, and Sexuality*. Berkeley, Los Angeles, London: University of California Press.

Hill, C. 2014. *Exposed: A History of Lingerie*. New Haven, London: Yale University Press in association with the Fashion Institute of Technology, New York.

Kyoto Costume Institute. 2002. *Fashion: A History from the 18th to the 20th Century*. Cologne: Taschen.

Lynn, E. 2010. *Underwear: Fashion in Detail*. London: Victoria & Albert Museum.

Smithsonian. 2012. *Fashion: The Definitive History of Costume and Style*. London, New York, Melbourne, Munich, Delhi: Dorling Kindersley.

Steele, V. 2001. *The Corset: A Cultural History*. New Haven, London: Yale University Press.

Waugh, N. 1954. *Corsets and Crinolines*. London, New York: Routledge/Theatre Art Books.

Acknowledgments

Thank you to my husband, Nick, for believing in me. You are the sun to my moon, and I love you more every day.

Thank you to my mother for giving me a love of reading and writing, for those weekly trips to the public library, and for passing on your love of beautiful things to me.

Thank you to my father for my sense of curiosity, for encouraging me to ask hard questions and seek honest answers, and for the set of encyclopedias in my childhood bedroom.

To my editor, Kaitlin, thank you for that very first email and for taking a risk on a brand-new author.

To my illustrator, Sandy, thank you for bringing this book to life. You were my first choice, and I am so incredibly grateful that you said yes.

To Angelina, Emma, Windy, Erin, and Dan, thank you for everything you've done to make this book a reality.

To Karolina and Keenan, thank you for lending your expertise.

To Krista, Quinne, Alysse, and Jason, thank you for keeping things running while I wrote this book. Everything would have been so much harder to do without you.

To Catherine, thank you for being my very first ally "in the industry." I am so proud to know you and to call you my friend.

To Santiago, Joe, and Karen, thank you. I wouldn't be who I am today without you.

To everyone who has ever supported *The Lingerie Addict*, thank you. You are the reason this book exists.

Index

Ten Speed Press and the Ten Speed Press colophon are registered
trademarks of Penguin Random House LLC.

Library of Congress Cataloging-in-Publication Data:
  Names: Harrington, Cora, author.
  Title: In intimate detail : how to choose, wear, and love lingerie / Cora
    Harrington.
  Description: First edition. | [Berkeley?] California : Ten Speed Press, 2018.
    | Includes bibliographical references and index.
  Identifiers: LCCN 2017041424
  Subjects: LCSH: Lingerie. | BISAC: DESIGN / Fashion. | HEALTH & FITNESS /
    Beauty & Grooming. | CRAFTS & HOBBIES / Fashion.
  Classification: LCC TT670 .H37 2018 | DDC 646/.34—dc23
  LC record available at https://lccn.loc.gov/2017041424

Hardcover ISBN: 978-0-399-58063-5
eBook ISBN: 978-0-399-58064-2

Printed in China

Design by Angelina Cheney
Illustrations by Sandy Wirt

10 9 8 7 6 5 4 3 2 1

First Edition